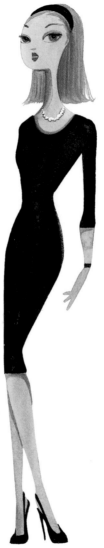

THE
LITTLE
BLACK
BOOK
OF
STYLE

Nina Garcia

ILLUSTRATIONS BY RUBEN TOLEDO

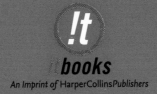

!t
it books
An Imprint of HarperCollinsPublishers

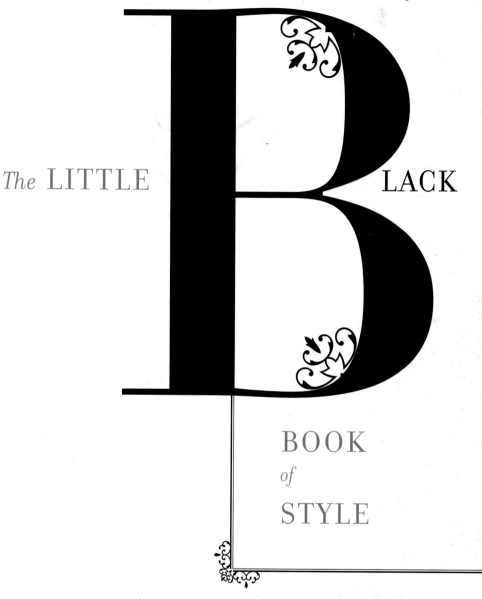

The LITTLE **B**LACK

BOOK

of

STYLE

A hardcover edition of this book was published in 2007 by Collins Living, an imprint of HarperCollins Publishers.

HarperCollins books may be purchased for educational, business, or sales promotional use. For information, please write: Special Markets Department, HarperCollins Publishers, 10 East 53rd Street, New York, NY 10022.

First It Books paperback published 2010.

Book design by Shubhani Sarkar

Library of Congress Cataloging-in-Publication data has been applied for.

ISBN 978-0-06-123721-8

10   11   12   13   14   ID/SCP   10   9   8   7   6   5   4   3   2   1

Inspiration gives no warnings.

GABRIEL GARCÍA MÁRQUEZ

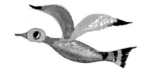

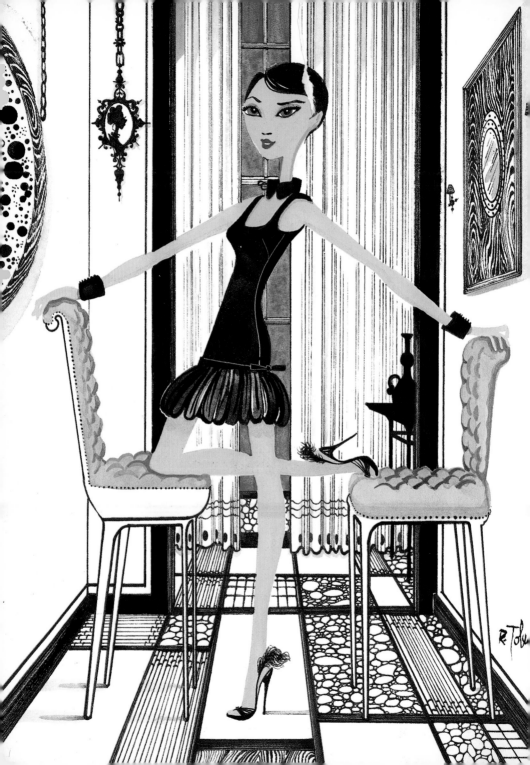

Contents

Preface

I GREW UP IN AN unbearably hot city on the northwest tip of Colombia, a place where style and art were part of the culture. I was constantly surrounded by incredibly vibrant, confident, feminine women, women who knew who they were and what image they wanted to convey to the world. They knew how to buy the right clothes for their bodies, how to edit out what did not suit them, and how to stay away from fads and maintain an aura of eternal style. It is my purpose with this book to inspire you the way these women inspired me.

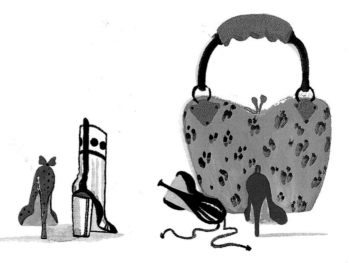

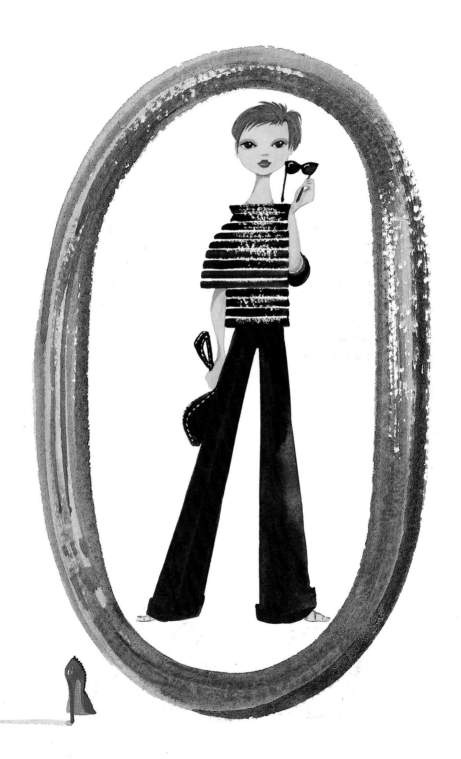

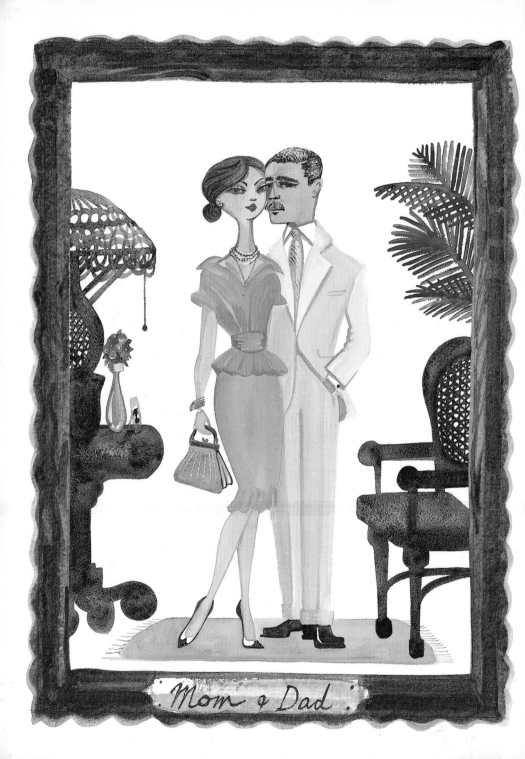

Mom & Dad

Author's Note

IN THE MORNINGS IN BARRANQUILLA, I would sit on my mother's closet floor and watch her. My mother was the kind of woman who gave the seamstress the key to our house (and later convinced her to move in), but kept her closet door locked at all times. Her closet was enormous, extraordinary, and off-limits—nobody was to go in there without her. Every piece of clothing was meticulously cared for, and I was not to touch anything. Each dress, skirt, and shirt was perfectly altered to suit her body and she would change them, adding sleeves, raising hemlines, to make them her own. My mother's closet revealed who she was: elegant, a frustrated actress, and a woman obsessed. She had to have her hair done every day; she refused to leave the house without lipstick; Lord knows how many plastic surgeries she had. As a child, I never understood why she cared so much.

My father was incredibly charming and incredibly handsome, and such a player. He had the power to make me think that white linen was the only fabric a man should wear. It was unrelentingly hot in our industrial town near the equator; to stay comfortable, my father wore only white linen pants and white guayaberas (linen shirts from Cuba). Every day I would watch him leave for work in that same outfit, and every day I thought he looked amazing. He was obsessed with traveling (my parents were quite an obsessive couple). My parents would take me out of school for weeks at a time and we would go around the world. Japan, India, France, Italy. My father always took us somewhere cold during the winter months, usually to the mountains skiing with a stop in New York or Paris. Since so much of my father's time was spent in the oppressive heat and humidity of Barranquilla, he really seemed infatuated with winter. On all of these trips, I learned about the culture, the fashions, the art, but most of all how differently everyone dressed. When we returned home, my mother would have piles of new clothes in need of alteration. My father would change back into his white linens and head to work. And I would return to school in the newest Parisian fashions, but a month behind on long division. I would complain to my father, who was much less concerned about it than I was. "But you saw the world," he would say. "There's always time to get caught up on long division!"

When I was fifteen, my parents sent me to an all-girls boarding school in Wellesley, Massachusetts. I strutted onto campus in a short skirt, high heels, and rabbit fur. There I stood, surrounded by khakis, jeans, pastel cable-knit sweaters, ribbon belts. "Look at the Colombian princess," the American girls must have been thinking. "We're gonna eat this one for lunch." I looked around this little bubble of preppiness. The girls all played lacrosse and they all dressed the same, more like boys than girls. I remember thinking, "Where the hell am I?" Before this moment, I considered myself really American and I thought I had seen everything. I had been to New York, Paris, Rome, but I had never seen this thing they called "preppy." But there I was, in maybe the preppiest town in America, nearly hyperventilating from my first experience with culture shock.

My mother took me into the Wellesley town center to see if we could find something that would help me blend in a bit. The only item I found somewhat appealing was a pink angora cardigan with pearl buttons (I know). I regretted the purchase almost immediately and the cardigan was soon stuffed into the far depths of my closet, never to be worn again. I decided to hold my own—I was not going to be intimidated, especially by girls who wore L.L. Bean duck boots.

Nothing can prepare a Colombian girl for the sight of one hundred American girls trudging across campus in duck boots. I'm sure I thought myself quite superior, but now I admire a lot of those very American things. I think that blue jeans and a white shirt can be the most fabulous outfit. It's all about how you wear it. And I love a Chanel bag, but I also see the perfection in an L.L. Bean canvas tote. Functional, chic, simple. It's about how you carry it. So I am proud to say that I owe a lot of my style to a strong, colorful Colombian woman, who taught me that how you present yourself to the world is important. And I owe a lot to a man in white linen who shunned mathematics and instead pushed me to see the world. And I also owe quite a bit to a group of American prep school girls, who gave me my first culture shock, who gave me the opportunity to hold my own, and who understood simplicity long before I did (though I'm still not sure about those boots).

Fashion fades, style is eternal.

COCO CHANEL

This book will change your life. Okay, maybe that's a bit dramatic. Maybe it won't change your life. But it will change your closet, which will in turn change your attitude, which can in fact change your life. So maybe it's not a bit dramatic. You be the judge.

This is not a book of rules. It is a book on style. I am not going to tell you when to wear white pants or when not to wear sandals. Instead, I am going to help you build your style confidence, find what works for you, edit your closet, teach you what to look for, and give you a few tricks of the trade. This is a crash course on style references, insider tips, and avoiding being the fashion victim. With this book I offer my own insights, a smattering of suggestions, some personal philosophies, and a bit of history. I hope to help simplify your approach to personal style by helping you build a foundation, cultivated through the perspective of a fashion editor who has already done the legwork (years of fashion shows and Ambien-aided flights . . . oh, you're welcome).

This book is meant to awaken the fashion editor inside you and help you decide what image you want to convey to the world. Above all, *The Little Black Book of Style* is meant to inspire you and make style fun. And if it changes your life along the way, well, don't say I never did anything for you.

Nina

THE
LITTLE
BLACK
BOOK
OF
STYLE

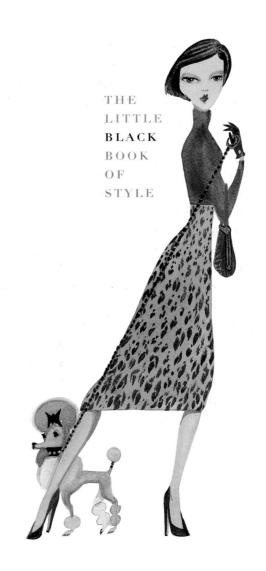

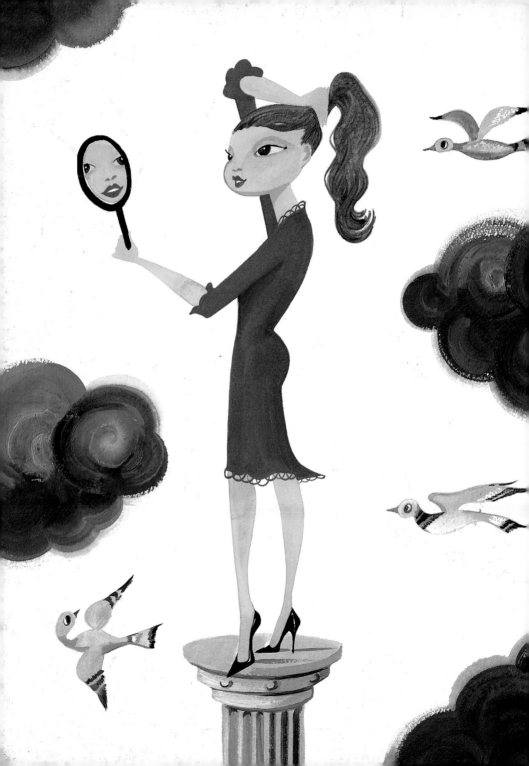

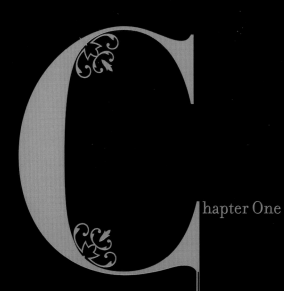

Chapter One

BE YOUR OWN MUSE

"Nothing makes
a woman more
beautiful than
the belief that
she is beautiful."

SOPHIA LOREN

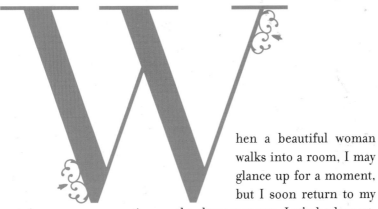

hen a beautiful woman walks into a room, I may glance up for a moment, but I soon return to my entrée or my conversation or the dessert menu. Let's be honest: beauty is not all that interesting (and certainly not more interesting than the dessert menu). But when a confident woman walks into a room, it is entrancing. I'll watch as she moves with poise and self-possession. She is not usually the one in the plain black dress. She is the one in the interesting shirt and the vintage skirt, and I immediately want to know where she got them. And she may not be the most stunningly gorgeous woman I've ever seen, but she has a way about her that can make her one of the most intriguing. Confidence is captivating, it is powerful, and it does not fade—and that is endlessly more interesting than beauty.

The first and most important step to developing style is to project this kind of confidence. The kind of confidence that tells others that you respect yourself, love yourself, and dress up for yourself and nobody else. You are your own muse. Style comes from knowing who you are and who you want to be in the world; it does not come from wanting to be somebody else, or wanting to be thinner, shorter, taller, prettier. Many of the most stylish women in the world have not been great beauties, but they have all drawn from an enormous amount of self-confidence. They made us think they were beautiful simply by believing it themselves. They did not let anyone else define them; they defined themselves.

I truly admire women who love themselves, even if they are not the standard beauty norm. I am fascinated by the "imperfect icons," the girls who are by far not the most beautiful girls in the room, but they are confident and think they're beautiful, so others think they are. I marvel at a six-foot-tall woman in stilettos, a big-bottomed woman in a curve-hugging skirt, a flat-chested woman in a tight, low cut T-shirt. When a woman embraces her "imperfections," they can become her greatest strengths, definers of her character and spirit. When she plays up her weaknesses and draws you to her flaws, she makes them special, attractive, and even enviable.

Confidence has nothing to do with aesthetics and everything to do with attitude. Nothing suits a woman better than this air of self-assurance, and when she truly owns that, she is unyielding and stunning. Confidence is the one thing that can instantly turn the volume up on a woman's beauty. When it comes to style and confidence, you have to learn to move with it, which can be daunting. We all have our insecurities. But you just know when you are in the company of a confident woman. Even (or especially) in the face of imperfections, her air is striking. Her beauty is fueled from something inside her. It's not that she doesn't care about her looks; on the contrary, she is so comfortable with who she is that she even embraces her quirks and flaws.

The confident woman loves herself entirely. Think Lauren Hutton and her gap-toothed smile. Think Frida Kahlo and her unibrow. Think the Duchess of Windsor, no great beauty. Think Barbra Streisand and her Grecian nose. Notice how their heads are always held up high and their flaws are always flaunted, never hidden or apologized for. Look to these women. Follow their lead. Hold your head up high and flaunt your flaws—the confidence should follow. And if all else fails, fake it. Confidence is the one thing that you can fake and you will actually end up believing it (oh, if that were true in other arenas!). You have to put yourself up on a pedestal before anyone is going to look up to you.

You are the goddess, so start treating yourself accordingly. Get your nails and hair done, take long baths, wear great perfume. Do whatever it is that makes you feel amazing. You have to pamper yourself, because nobody else is going to do it for you. Start adoring yourself. Love yourself from the inside out, and slowly but surely you will become comfortable on that pedestal, and you will exude the kind of confidence that others admire. And what you wear up on that pedestal matters. Sweatsuits just won't do. I promise you, a great dress or a stunning skirt will make you feel much more "spotlight worthy," and others will see you that way too.

What you wear is how you present yourself to the world, especially today, when human contacts are so quick. Fashion is instant language.

MIUCCIA PRADA

This instant language is much smarter than it gets credit for at times. They are just clothes, shoes, and bags, you could say. And people do say it, day after day. But I think they are more than just clothes, shoes, and bags. They are a large part of a woman's character and tell us a bit of her story without saying a word.

It was also Miuccia Prada who said, "I thought fashion was stupid because I thought there were more intelligent and noble professions, like politics, medicine, or science." And I think every woman has this hesitation at one time or another. I did. I spent four years of college trying to find out what I wanted to do that did not involve the fashion industry. But I always came back to it. And not for the free samples (they are not as free as you might think). I came back to it because I was in love with style, and I finally recognized it as something important and influential.

I have always found that the women with amazing personal style are powerful, intriguing, and yes, even intelligent. Very intelligent. They know who they are and what they want to project upon the world. These women understand that what they put on in the morning is the first thing that people notice about them. It tells the world a bit of their story. And, more important, their clothes affect how they feel about themselves throughout the day.

Think about this when you stand in front of your closet in the morning contemplating those safe choices (ugh), those trendy choices (ugh), and those choices that tell the world who you are (yes). When you choose according to you inner muse, you will project an aura of confidence and self-assuredness that nobody else can touch.

And once you've got confidence, the rest is gravy.

I was not ugly. I might never be anything for men to lose their heads about, but I need never again be ugly. This knowledge was like a song within me. Suddenly it all came together. If you were healthy, fit, and well-dressed, you could be attractive.

ELSIE DE WOLFE

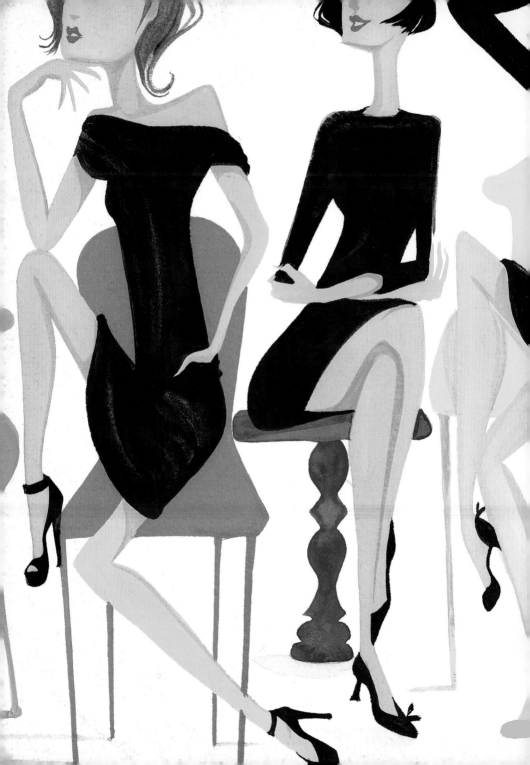

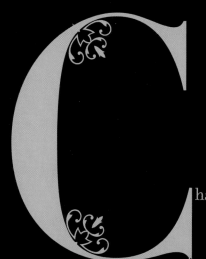

Chapter Two

THE BASICS

"Fashion can be bought. Style one must possess."

EDNA WOOLMAN CHASE

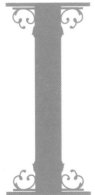

t is truly unique when you see that one girl who is so different, the one who you just have to walk up to and ask her about her skirt, shirt, bag, etc. I don't see that girl nearly as often as I would like. Be that girl. Anyone can be "in fashion," all one has to do is follow the herd and abide by the rules of the season. But style is personal. There is no herd to follow. There are no rules. There are no seasons. Style comes from within. If there is anything absolute about style, it is that it holds you accountable to yourself at every moment. You have to be confident with who you are on the inside before you can ever fully be comfortable presenting yourself to the outside world. And how you present yourself to the world is important. It is inherently related to your sense of self. Every time you dress you assert some aspect of yourself and your identity. With style, you tell the world who you are, or at least the story of who you would like to be on that particular day. Style affords you opportunities. It opens doors and allows you the chance to showcase a facet of yourself in an obvious and inimitable way.

A stylish woman makes me want to walk up to her and say "Where did you get that?" It is not in any magazine or on any runway I have seen, and I just have to find out where it is from. A flea market, her grandmother's closet, wherever. I just know that I have not seen it before, which is the most intriguing thing in the world. All of the great style icons achieved this aura of intrigue. They were the first to step on the scene with clothes and accessories that left the rest of the world asking, "Where did she get that?' Because style icons never follow the leader, they never abide by rules.

I have spent ten years at *Elle*, six as the fashion director. In all this time, I have been to countless fashion shows, seen trends fade in and out, watched stylish women come and go, designers rise and fall. I have been surrounded by the fashionable and the fantastic, and I have learned that there are a few very basic guidelines (ten, in my book) that all of these fashionable and fantastic people know. I'm going to give them to you straight, because when it comes to style, there are no rules, as the cliché goes, but there are definite basics. A true style icon breaks the rules and ignores the trends, but she has these ten basics down pat:

A STYLE ICON KNOWS

- HOW TO EDIT. She only buys what she likes and what looks good on her.
- TO INVEST IN "THE BONES" (the classic trench, the little black dress . . .) and builds from there.
- TO BUY WITH DRAMA. She goes for that over-the-top, decadent item. If she falls in love, she takes it home.
- THE UTMOST IMPORTANCE OF SHOES. Lots of shoes.
- AND THE POWER OF ACCESSORIES. Done just the right way.
- A GOOD TAILOR.

- HOW NOT TO BE THE FASHION VICTIM. She never buys into the trends and she never carries the "it" bag.
- IT IS NOT ABOUT THE MONEY. She wears her flea market Mexican earrings the same way she would wear her diamonds.
- HOW TO MIX IT UP.
- HOW TO BE IMPERFECT. She understands that every day is not a photo shoot.

And that is style.

BASIC #1
How to edit

I am constantly editing and searching for just the right pieces to put on the pages of the magazine. Season after season, I head to the fashion shows in New York, Paris, Milan, and London, picking out the most important accessories and clothing. I scour through hundreds upon hundreds of pieces, looking for the truly remarkable and editing out all that is not utterly amazing. I want you to do this with your closet. Be an editor. Your closet should only contain amazing choices—it is much easier to be inspired when you see five remarkable pieces than when you see twenty-five pieces and twenty of them are unremarkable. Pick out those key items and get rid of the rest.

I don't care if it is the latest trend or the "must-have" item of the season. I don't care if you spent a week's salary on it in 1999 so that you could afford it. I don't care if you wore it every day in

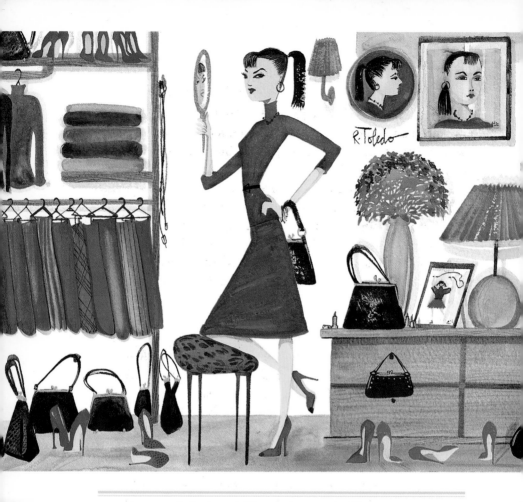

"I love America, and I love American women,
but there is one thing that deeply shocks me . . .
American closets. I cannot believe one can
dress well when you have so much.

ANDRÉE PUTMAN

college and you "can't bear to part with it." If it doesn't look good on you, it should not be in your closet. Why are you holding on to those jeans from high school? Why are you holding on to those hot pink hot pants (seriously, why)?

Your closet is probably bursting at the seams, but how many items in there do you actually wear? How many of those items make you feel good about yourself? And how many times have you looked in that closet and said, "I have nothing to wear!"? Mornings are rough enough; help yourself out a little bit. Edit your closet, then edit your shopping habits, and I promise you that being stylish will become much easier.

- THROW OUT WHAT YOU DON'T WEAR AND WHAT DOESN'T LOOK GOOD ON YOU. So simple to say, yet so hard follow through on. So make yourself a deal. For every twenty items you toss, you can buy one killer piece.
- BUY THE RIGHT SIZE. If you are a size 8, do not buy a size 6 "because you are going to lose weight." It is better to buy the realistic size and enjoy the way the clothes make you feel at that moment. And really, who wants a too-tight pair of pants in their closet to taunt them every day? I much prefer to be seduced by chocolate and a pair of pants that flatters me.
- DON'T BE SUCKED IN BY THE SALE TAG. Paying $100 for a pair of jeans that cost $200 is a great deal. But if you are never going to wear those jeans, you don't need them, or really even like them, that's a very expensive deal.
- DON'T PLAY IT TOO SAFE. A closet full of safe choices is no fun. And fashion should be fun! You should wake up in

the morning and be inspired by what is in your closet, and twenty black skirts tend to offer little inspiration. One white beaded vintage skirt offers a lot.

- DO NOT BUY ACCORDING TO THE TRENDS. This drives me crazy. If the trend is to wear bright yellow mini-dresses and you don't look good in yellow or mini-dresses, why would you buy one? Wear what suits you and what makes you comfortable.
- BE RUTHLESS WHEN YOU EDIT. Do not keep items in your closet for sentimental reasons. If you absolutely cannot get rid of that old jean jacket you used to wear, put it in storage and revisit it years later (when you are heading to a costume party). Do not keep items just because you paid a lot for them. Or because you'll fit into them again one fine day. Or because you think they are beautiful, but just don't look good on you. Let them go! Pass them down to someone who will wear them. If you haven't worn them in years, you will never wear them again. Your closet should be full of only pieces that look good on you and make you feel good about yourself. Your skinny jeans from high school? That trendy dress that you've never worn? I promise you, you won't miss them.

And now you're ready to begin.

The more you know, the less you need.

ABORIGINAL SAYING

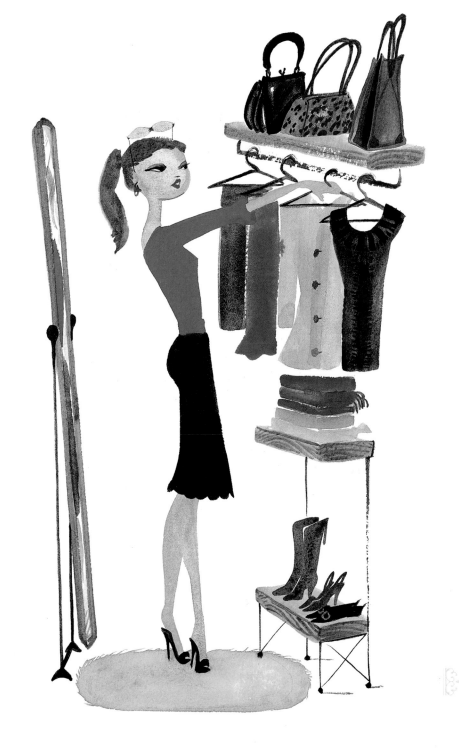

BASIC #2
Invest in the bones

The bones of your wardrobe are those essential staples that go with almost anything, never go out of style, and are enduringly chic. They are meant to be a blank canvas that you can layer on to. They are dependable and perhaps unremarkable, but a stylish woman understands that not every piece is supposed to be remarkable. Some items are just supposed to be reliable.

These ten staples transcend time, trends, and travel. They can go from day to night, season to season, and they can still be worn five years from now. They should supersede any fads—don't buy the trendy versions—these are the classics. And they work just as well in New York, Paris, Tokyo, and Sydney.

The Little Black Dress

The ultimate blank canvas. It is mysterious and chic, understated and provocative. In its simplicity, it makes you look effortlessly stylish. In its sophistication, it makes you look endlessly elegant. The little black dress is the dress that is going to let you shine—it is going to flatter you, but it is not going to detract from the rest of you. It lets your hair, your accessories, and your personality take center stage. And the slimming effect—let's not forget the slimming effect.

THE TEST OF TIME: Fashion legend has it that Coco Chanel created the first little black dress. It represents all that Chanel stood for: comfort, practicality, and self-assured sexiness. But fashion legends always try to be associated with Coco Chanel. In fact, the LBD was not the brainchild of the brilliant French designer, it was simply born out of practicality. Years before Chanel debuted her LBD, the gar-

> *One is never over- or underdressed*
> *with a little black dress.*
>
> KARL LAGERFELD

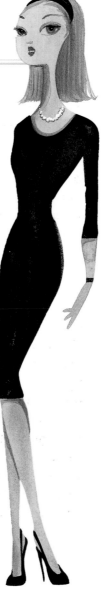

ment had found its way into women's closets. As women grew busier, they needed stylish items that were also versatile, comfortable, and practical. The little black dress emerged as a product of necessity. But, yes, it was Chanel who perpetuated the legend in 1926, when she debuted her famous "Ford" design, which to this day remains an item that is elegant, seductive, flattering, and practical.

A classic men's white shirt

The classic white shirt is as key to American style as blue jeans. It is chic and simple. Practical and unpretentious. It can be paired with jeans (Jackie O. in Hyannis), black pants (Uma Thurman in *Pulp Fiction*), a long skirt (Audrey Hepburn in *Roman Holiday*), a gown (Sharon Stone on the red carpet). It is also incredibly useful to cover up a bad outfit when entering a good hotel (Julia Roberts in *Pretty Woman*).

THE TEST OF TIME: Nobody knows who the first woman to throw on the man's shirt was, but she is the kind of woman I'd like to meet. You know she understood the appeal of effortlessness and a

*The Alpha and the Omega of the
fashion alphabet. The creative universe begins
with its essentiality and, whatever path the
imagination takes, ends with its purity.*

GIORGIO ARMANI

complete lack of pretension. As early as the 1920s, during the birth of the garçonne look, women were photographed in men's shirts. In the 1950s, Audrey Hepburn liked to wear a man's shirt and tie the tails twice around her tiny waist. In 1977, Diane Keaton's eponymous character in Annie Hall wore the shirt, several sizes too large—and incited a craze. And in 1998, Sharon Stone stepped onto the red carpet in a lavender Vera Wang skirt and her husband's white shirt, tied back with a dragonfly pin. Don't say you weren't impressed. The white shirt has endured decade after decade. Any time a cool girl or a designer throws a man's shirt into the mix, we are reminded of the power that comes with that crisp simplicity. And is there anything quite so sensual as seeing a woman in a man's white shirt?

I do not believe in God. I believe in cashmere.

FRAN LEBOWITZ

Cashmere cardigan or turtleneck

In all kinds of weather and for any kind of occasion, throwing on cashmere makes you feel instantly luxe. The first time you try it on, you immediately understand what all the fuss is about. A cashmere cardigan is perfect over anything—a dress, a T-shirt, a button-down shirt—but also incredibly sexy when worn alone, à la Marilyn Monroe. A turtleneck is also perfect paired with most everything—jeans, trousers, skirts.

THE TEST OF TIME: Sweaters came to prominence in the 1890s when men and women wore them for sports and equestrian activities, though before World War I they were bulky and not all that attractive. One brisk day on a polo field, Coco Chanel borrowed a player's jersey, belted it, and found that she quite liked the look. She started to make similar sweaters, which were soon snatched up by her customers. In 1937, the sweater got its biggest boost when Lana Turner wore a very tight, form-fitting sweater in the 1937 film *They Won't Forget*. She is only on the screen briefly as she walks down the street of a Southern town in that sweater, but it was an influential walk. Turner would forever be known as "the sweater girl," and women the world over became sweater girls too.

A trench coat

A classic trench can work in any kind of weather and goes well with almost anything (or almost nothing if you are feeling very film noir). But the best part of the trench coat is that it makes you instantly mysterious. Wear it with big sunglasses if you want to really channel your inner detective, spy, or fugitive.

THE TEST OF TIME: The trench coat was first created by Thomas Burberry for the British army officers in World War I. It was designed keep them warm and dry in the trenches (hence the name), and every element of the coat had a purpose. The waterproof fabric and removable wool lining made it serviceable in all weather; the epaulettes were originally used to hold gloves or service hats; the D-rings on the belt were made to secure grenades; the huge pockets were meant to hold maps and extra ammo. And though unnecessary today, these utilitarian details are maintained in the modern coat. Jean-Paul Gaultier and Yves Saint Laurent have made careers out of reinventing different versions of the trench, but the basic elements remain the same. The design has barely changed in ninety years, which is what makes the trench so glamorous and alluring.

Put on a trench, you're suddenly
Audrey Hepburn walking along the Seine.

MICHAEL KORS

I have often said that I wish I had invented blue jeans: the most spectacular, the most practical, the most relaxed and nonchalant. They have expression, modesty, sex appeal, simplicity—all I hope for in my clothes.

YVES SAINT LAURENT

Denim

There is something about jeans that gives a girl an aura of instant style. They are simple and practical. Sexy and perfect. Rebellious and elegant. They are the most versatile, most perfect item. The most alluring part about denim is that it can dress anything down and make even the most uptight items look relaxed.

For years, Nan Kempner was one of America's most stylish women, in large part because she understood the allure of mixing pieces (often denim pieces) in a very American way. Last year, The Met had an exhibit on Nan and the opening silhouette featured an elegant ball gown paired with one of Nan's classic denim shirts. It was so refreshing, and so utterly American. The jean made the ball gown seem practical, relaxed, casual, and so unassuming. This is the true power of denim.

THE TEST OF TIME: In the 1850s, Levi Strauss started selling rugged blue jeans to the gold miners in San Francisco, who needed pants that were durable and comfortable. In 1873, Jacob Davis, and a tailor from Reno, Nevada, contacted Strauss with the idea to rivet the pockets to make the design stronger; the two men went into business, patented the improved pants, and stepped into history. Today, over a hundred years since Strauss and Davis took out the patent, blue jeans have grown from being just a practical pair of pants to being one of the sexiest and seductive articles of clothing imaginable.

A man's classic watch

Women's watches tend to change according to trends, but a classic man's watch is timeless and looks great on a woman's wrist. It makes a statement and breaks the rules in an unexpected but subtle way. It's another great item to "borrow" from a boyfriend/husband/father/friend.

THE TEST OF TIME: Women first started to wear wristwatches in Europe in the 1880s, when they attached their pocket watches to leather wristbands to go out hunting or horseback riding. Soon enough the wristwatch began to be manufactured for women, but men stuck with the pocket watch and considered the new wristwatch style too effeminate. It was not until World War I, when the soldiers realized that the effeminate wristwatch actually might be a more efficient choice when being shot at by rapid fire. Almost overnight, European manufacturers started working overtime converting women's wristwatches into military timepieces. The man's watch was born—they were late to the game, but they do deserve credit for having some of the most classic designs. They stole it from us; it's quite alright (and quite satisfying) to steal it back.

Diamonds

You can't go wrong here. They are perfect for day or night, casual or dressy, winter or summer, with other jewels, or not. Fake is fine.

THE TEST OF TIME: In the fifteenth century, King Charles VII of France gave his mistress, Agnès Sorel, a diamond ring. Agnès took quite a liking to the stone and started to wear as many as possible, an understandable move. But it is a notable move because before Agnès, diamonds were strictly for men. They were a symbol of power, status, and valor, and women were legally not allowed to wear them. Agnès publicly defied French law and made it acceptable and fashionable for women to wear diamonds. Half a millennium later, there is no sign of the diamond going out of style.

Big girls need big diamonds.

ELIZABETH TAYLOR

Ballet flats

There are a few moments (very few) when you have to give your heels the boot in the name of practicality or shopping strategy. Let's review: 1) In an airport, when you may have to make mad dashes. 2) On the first day of the Barneys sale, when you will have to make mad dashes. 3) On sand, which is actually quite tragic because there is no better time for a high heel's boost than when you are half-naked. But the harsh reality is: Stilettos and sand just don't mix. 4) When driving. Even if you think you've mastered the technique, you have not. And insurance hikes can put a damper on a girl's shoe budget.

THE TEST OF TIME: When faced with these situations, a pair of ballet flats will help you through. Ballet flats, as the name suggests, were inspired by ballet dancers. They were introduced in France by Repetto, an American company that specialized in dance wear. Capezio, another American dance-wear company, ran with it and in 1949 created a pair of patent leather flats with ankle ribbons. In the 1950s designers began to create their own variations on the shoe, and actresses began wearing them on screen (Audrey Hepburn and Brigitte Bardot). Ballet flats became a staple in every woman's closet and have helped us navigate tricky terrain ever since.

A classic high-heel pump

I am a big supporter of buying outrageous, impractical, bold shoes. I also think that you should have at least one classic high-heel that you can rely on for those times when that fierce red patent leather stiletto won't do. While the red stiletto is just the kind of shoe you want to take out on the town, she's probably going to clash with a few outfits and most prospective in-laws. She's just that kinda shoe—that is, after all, why we love her. But you can't depend on the red stiletto the way you can depend on, say, a classic black high-heel pump. The red stiletto will get a lot more attention, but the black pump will let the other pieces of your outfit speak, which is sometimes just what you need from a shoe.

THE TEST OF TIME: Nobody knows who invented the high heel. Some credit Leonardo Da Vinci. Sure, I'll buy that. We do know that it dates back to at least 1533 when Catherine de Medici wore a two-inch heel for her wedding ceremony to make her appear taller. The world had to wait more than five hundred years for the stiletto to be born in the 1950s, but we have Catherine de Medici to thank for laying the two-inch groundwork on her wedding day.

A great bag

The bag, like the shoe, is a great place to have fun and play with colors, textures, and shapes. But, like the shoe, you should have at least one classic bag (okay, maybe three) that will go with you anywhere.

Every woman should have:

- A TOTE OR SHOULDER BAG: for daytime and carrying around almost everything.
- A CLUTCH: for nighttime and carrying around almost nothing.
- A MEDIUM-SIZED HANDBAG, WITH A CHAIN-LINK STRAP: for those times in between.
- THE MUST-HAVE BAG: Chanel 2.55, Louis Vuitton Speedy, Gucci's Jackie O., Hermès Birkin.

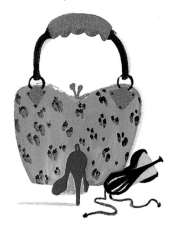

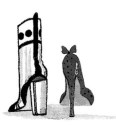

THE TEST OF TIME: The handbag only became a female accessory at the beginning of the 1900s. Before that only men carried a purse, and if a woman wanted something, she had to ask him for it. Women put an end to that at the turn of the twentieth century, when they started heading out in the world alone and carrying their own belongings, thank you very much. The handbag became a sign of independence, which is another reason you should not cower to the "it bag" syndrome (see "Basic #7: How not to be a fashion victim").

These items are timeless and unbelievably chic in their simplicity. They are your base, to which you can add just enough flair and funkiness to make them unbelievably stylish. They can be found at crazy, phenomenal prices, but also crazy, affordable prices. The cost does not matter here. What matters is that you buy them as classic as possible. They cannot be too trendy, too fussy, or too colorful. This is not where the drama is going to come from—this is your white canvas. The drama comes next.

Simplicity is the ultimate sophistication.

LEONARDO DA VINCI

Buy what is truly fantastic. The leopard-print coat, the knock-them-dead dress, the decadent piece of jewelry. You should spend your money on those one-of-a-kind, dramatic pieces. You know one when you see one. You fall in love with it immediately. Yes, it may cost you a small fortune, but it is worth it. You know you look good in it, everyone else knows you look good in it, and it is going to make you feel amazing. So go a little crazy.

But buy timeless items. Don't just go crazy for the trends. Make sure you can see yourself wearing it a few seasons later. You should not buy the trends with drama. Buying with drama usually involves dropping a bit of cash, and you should never drop a lot of cash on a passing fad. Make it a rule that when you spend a lot of money, you consider whether or not you will love it three, five, even ten years from now. Also consider if it reflects your personal style. It's like falling in love and going on that first date. You just know.

The best time to buy with drama is when you are traveling. Always pick something up that is exotic—some odd trapping that catches your eye at the market or from a street vendor. Nobody else is going to have it back home and it will be uniquely yours.

If you do happen to fall in love with a trend (it happens), it is far more interesting to buy it now and wait a few years until it is out of style to wear it. But maybe I'm the only crazy person who would do this.

Some dramatic pieces to go crazy for:

- AN OVERSIZE COCKTAIL RING: A great statement—or conversation piece. Also lovely to twirl around when incredibly bored at a cocktail party (which hardly ever happens. Right.).

- A KNOCK-'EM-DEAD EVENING OR COCKTAIL DRESS: You just need one. Invest the money in something truly amazing. A hand-beaded dress, a vintage forties dress, a dress that fits you perfectly. It may take you years to comb through sample sales, but find that dress.
- A CUFF: Yet another inherited accessory from Mme. Chanel. Wear one or two bejeweled or plain cuffs. They are always chic and sophisticated.
- A PIECE OF FUR: Adds a touch of luxury in the winter and for evening. If you want to go really dramatic, a fabulous fur coat will do too!
- KILLER SHOES: Go for high-heeled strappy sandals in metallic gold or silver.
- AN EXOTIC BAG: A croc bag that you fall in love with today will probably have the same appeal ten years from now.
- A STAND-OUT COAT: It is going to get a lot of mileage in the winter—it hardly matters what you are wearing underneath if the coat is fabulous.

Go a little crazy.
Be a little dramatic.
Have a lot of fun.

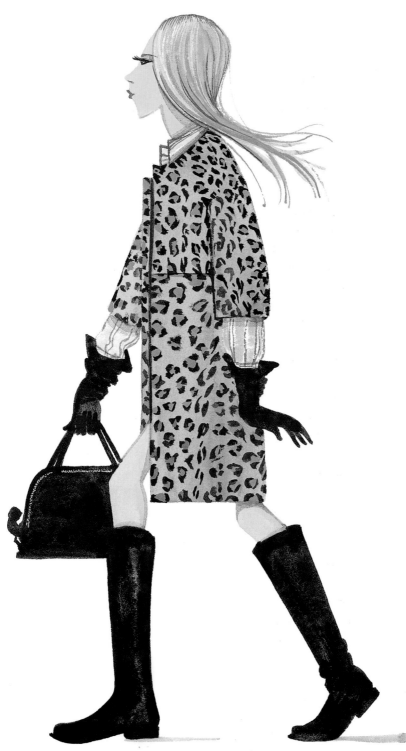

TOLEDO

Give a girl the right shoes and
she can conquer the world.

BETTE MIDLER

You can never have enough high heels. You just can't. People will try to tell you differently. Smile politely and slowly strut away. A great pair of heels is a powerful thing—it can change your mood, your posture, and your attitude; it can make a boring outfit instantly fabulous, and it always makes your legs look better. How many things in the world have that much power? I don't know of any. This is why I respect the shoe and often start the entire dressing process with the shoe and let it inspire the rest of my look.

Disclaimer: I know I said there are no rules when it comes to style, but we are talking shoes here. It's a whole different ball game and I feel it necessary to lay down the ground rules:

Invest in a good pair of shoes

Even if it's only one pair. There are only a few designers who make very good shoes. It is difficult and expensive to make a perfect, quality shoe. It is also impossible to make a cheap shoe look expensive. Spend wisely here, because it really matters. The names that you hear repeatedly have certainly earned their reputation, among them:

- MANOLO BLAHNIK: The sexiest and the safest investment. A sure thing.
- CHRISTIAN LOUBOUTIN: To-die-for red soles, the most creative styles, big on toe cleavage.
- ROGER VIVIER: Extremely chic and one-of-a-kind.
- JIMMY CHOO: Very sexy and the most comfortable. For the real chameleon.
- AZZEDINE ALAÏA: For the connoisseur and adventuress.

Wear your size

Often in my business, I see fashionistas who are a size 7 try to fit into a sample size 9. I guess they think that nobody will notice. People notice. And when girls try to squeeze into a smaller size, the effect is ghastly. Toes spilling out of a pair of strappy, sexy sandals is a very painful sight. I do not wince out of sympathy for your feet. I side with the shoe.

Only show two cracks

Toe cleavage does not get the attention it deserves, but trust me, it matters. Two cracks, no more.

Get pedicures

Chipped toe polish, cracked heels, etc. are not acceptable.

Don't go too high

I am a fan of height, but there is such a thing as too high (over four inches). You will not be able to walk correctly in a heel over four inches. Your posture will shift and you will look ridiculous!

Watch your proportions

Hardly anyone can pull off a very short skirt with a very high heel without looking like a tramp.

You can never have enough high heels

Never.

I did not have three thousand pairs of shoes,
I had one thousand and sixty.

IMELDA MARCOS

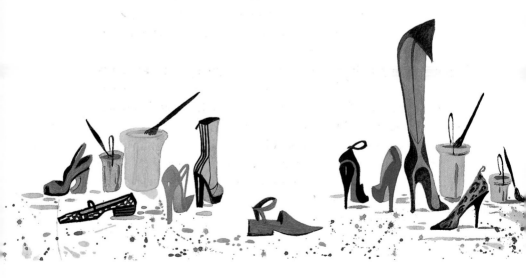

Those miniskirts, that slinky dress, your skinny jeans. Gain ten pounds and they betray you in a heartbeat, the cows. But your accessories—your shoes and bags, your scarves and necklaces. They'll stand by you through thick and thin. They don't care if you gain twenty pounds, they'll hang right there with you. They will always make you feel better about yourself. They will pull together an outfit for you. They will help you update your wardrobe without spending a ton of money. And, without saying a word, they'll spend all day talking you up to the world, telling others how cool, fun, elegant, and sophisticated you are. Really, what else can you ask for in a friend?

Stylish women know how to cozy up to an accessory. Jackie O. and her sunglasses. Audrey Hepburn and her scarf. Elizabeth Taylor and her diamonds. These women understood that you didn't have to wear an outlandish dress if you invited your best accessories to the party. Aristotle Onassis once said of Jackie, "I don't know what she does with all the clothes she buys. I only ever see her in blue jeans." Yes, but she wore those blue jeans with perfect Saint Tropez sandals and signature shades and she became instantly chic. And Audrey Hepburn is forever immortalized by her simplicity (the black pants and turtleneck, the sleeveless dresses), but it was the scarf that she tied every which way (around her neck, her hat, her head, her waist) that set her apart. And Elizabeth Taylor (if we forgive her those *Dynasty* days) mostly wore an elegant black or white sleeveless dress and let her jewels announce her arrival . . . or engagement. Her seven marriages may have ended, but the woman never let go of her jewels. This is a dame we can learn from.

A woman's relationship with her accessories is important and elemental. She should choose her accessories as she chooses her friends, seeking out the ones that complement who she is, let her have fun, make her feel confident when she walks down the street, and stick by her through her ups and downs, her men, and her extra pounds. Because your accessories, like your friends, tell the world who you are.

The key to accessorizing is to keep it personal and to keep it tasteful. To make it personal, wear something that means something to you: Grandmother's old cross pendant or an antique watch or a bracelet from Mexico. And to be tasteful, make sure you don't go overboard. If you have on a big necklace and big earrings, take one off. Limit it to one. Too much of a good thing can turn into a bad thing very quickly.

The only thing that separates us from the animals is our ability to accessorize.

OLYMPIA DUKAKIS IN *STEEL MAGNOLIAS*

Once you find a good tailor, do not give away his name, not even under the threat of bodily harm.

A GOOD YEAR

A good tailor is like a good pair of shoes—necessary, worth every penny, and capable of making you look ten pounds thinner. Find a good tailor. Make friends with him. Buy him gifts during the holidays. Ask him about his family. Compliment him on his work. Tip him well. A good tailor is one of the most important people in your life. I know you may be thinking I'm being a bit dramatic about this. And true, I was raised by a woman who convinced her seamstress to move into our house, but I now understand the method to my mother's madness (if a spare bedroom in Manhattan wasn't so damn expensive . . .).

I used to watch in fascination as my mother and her seamstress would transform articles of clothing. They didn't just take the clothes in to fit my mother's body, they would also change the design around—adding sleeves, raising hemlines, elongating dresses—so that each item was customized to my mother's style. I have come to appreciate just how invaluable a good tailor or seamstress is.

Before you go to the tailor, it helps if you study a few designer pieces (in the dressing room is fine). Look at the cuts and the seams, notice how certain designs make you look taller, thinner, and more polished. Then, when you go to the tailor, you will know exactly what to ask of them.

Clothes make the man. Naked people have little or no influence on society.

A good tailor can:
- make any piece of clothing look expensive (an ill-fitting designer jacket looks cheaper than a perfectly tailored hand-me-down).
- fit clothes to your body without changing the look or shape.
- revive older items (a blazer from the eighties can be revamped to look chic and modern with the right alterations).
- shorten your pant legs, but maintain the same hem style (especially important when it comes to jeans).
- turn your vintage finds into one-of-a-kind keepsakes.
- rework a fur coat (your mother's or grandmother's) and make it completely new.
- make anything you want. If you have an amazing imagination and an amazing tailor, you can have him make that one perfect item that you want. That's my personal dream. I'm still looking for that tailor.

How to find a good tailor:

- ask your (well-dressed) friends.
- ask the salespeople at the high-end boutiques.
- don't be afraid to ask questions.
- test him/her out with a simple job first.

BASIC #7
How not to be a fashion victim

Every time I see a woman with the "it bag" du jour I do not envy her; I pity her, the poor thing. She just dropped ten grand to look like a wannabe. The "it bag" is something I will never understand. Why would someone want to carry around a bag that advertises "Fashion Victim"? It's like carrying around a white flag of surrender—a rather expensive white flag of surrender, usually made of black leather. The "it bag" is not going to set your wardrobe apart or make any unique style statement, and the bag is where you should have a little fun. Find one in red or patent leather—anything that speaks to your style and doesn't make you look like a lemming. Lemmings are not cute.

Only dead fish swim with the stream.

MALCOLM MUGGERIDGE

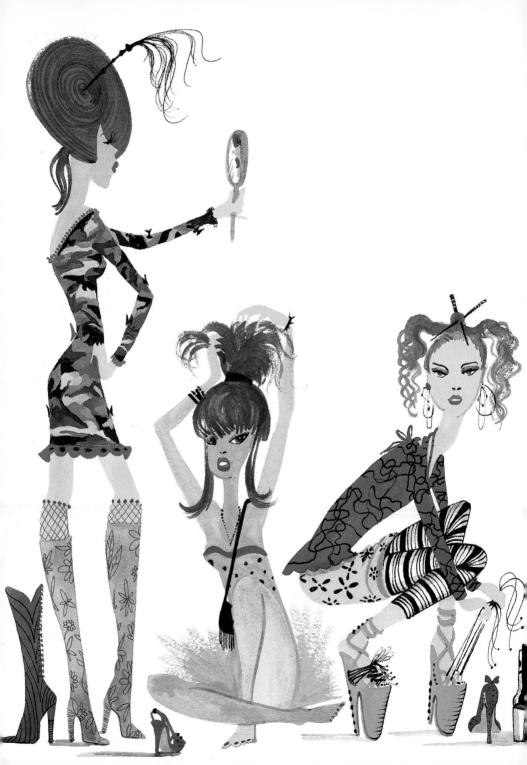

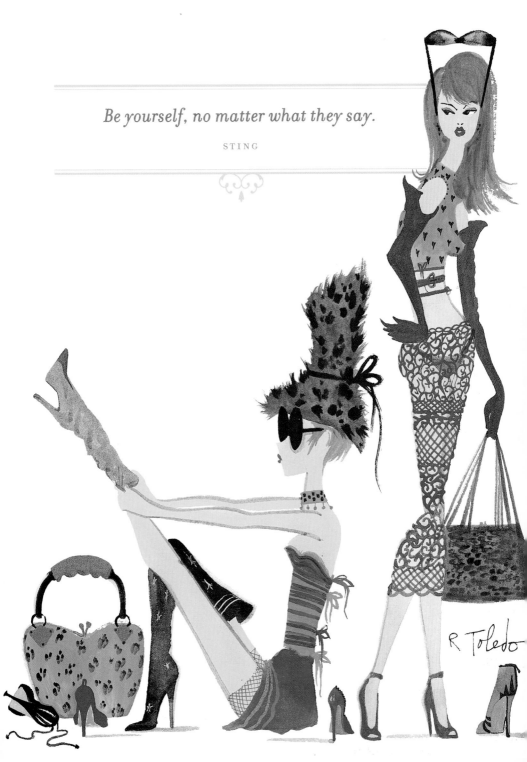

Be yourself, no matter what they say.

STING

Another way to spot a fashion victim (besides the "it bag" flag) is to count the designer pieces she is wearing. She'll usually help you out by putting the labels on conspicuous display. But you can just walk up to her and ask. She'll proudly tell you; "Prada, Gucci, Chanel." I'm willing to bet she's not wearing any H&M; the poor girl has not yet been enlightened. [Disclaimer: I'm not knocking Prada, Gucci, or Chanel (or Hermès, for that matter)—I'm not dumb. I love Prada, Gucci, and Chanel (and Hermès for that matter)—see, I'm actually quite smart. But I am knocking buying Prada, Gucci, and Chanel, (or Hermès) just because it's the trendy thing to do.]

A third way to spot a fashion victim (this one's a bit harder and takes some practice) is to note how many of her clothing choices were inspired by the season's trends. One trend—a great piece of trendy turquoise jewelry, perhaps—is lovely. Two trends—the turquoise necklace and maybe the newest skirt style—can be quite lovely too. Three trends and we start entering dangerous territory. The necklace, the skirt, and the latest corked stiletto, and flares start to go off. Four trends—the necklace, the skirt, the stiletto, and the must-have ruffle-trim top—and the victim is pretty much a done deal.

It's not money that makes you well-dressed,
it's understanding.

CHRISTIAN DIOR

Fashion is expensive. Style is not. Some of the most stylish girls I know are certainly not the wealthiest. Ironically, it is often the girls with less money who seem to understand style the best. Maybe it's because they are forced to be picky and cannot slavishly follow the trends. Maybe it's because they consider their purchases more carefully. Maybe it's because they have perfected the art of mixing their more expensive items with their cheaper finds. Or maybe it's because they know where to splurge and where to save.

Every once in a while a wealthy icon reminds us how great a cheap thrill can be. Kate Moss caused a stir when she was photographed carrying a £2.99 bag from Superdrug. Within hours, sales increased tenfold.

Cheap thrills:

- WHITE HANES T-SHIRTS: Laid-back and great for mixing. Best when taken from your boyfriend's or husband's drawer.
- L. L. BEAN TOTE: Simple, chic, and functional.
- A WHITE BUTTON-UP: Will go with anything.
- KHAKI PANTS: Perfectly classic. Just don't go pleated.
- FLEA-MARKET FINDS: If you love it, haggle for it. A general rule of thumb is to offer three times less than you want to pay.
- ANYTHING H&M, TARGET, UNIQLO: First-rate style at cut-rate prices.
- VINTAGE STEALS: Cheapest when taken from your mother's closet.

Anything that sounds like it won't make sense usually looks amazing. The uptown with the downtown. The soft with the hard. The casual with the elegant. Trust me, it works. Unpredictable is far more interesting than predictable. It is what is going to make you look different and interesting, which is the hallmark of a stylish woman. Mixing it up is not about looking staged. It is supposed to be personal. Keep those items that are uniquely you.

Mixing it up means taking the unexpected and making it yours. I had never been an old-lady-diamond-bracelet kind of girl. I just didn't see the appeal. But at a dinner party one night, this incredibly chic and stylish woman was wearing one of these old lady bracelets. She paired it with her beads from Thailand, her Kabbalah string, and a few other pieces that she never takes off. She made it a part of who she was, and for the first time in my life, I wanted an old lady diamond bracelet . . . or maybe I was just in awe of the expert mix-and-match situation. I never got the bracelet, but I never forgot the image of that perfectly imperfect mix.

Style is about these imperfect mixes and these unusual juxtapositions, it takes time and trial to perfect the mix. It can't look staged, it has to look effortless.

*The world just does not fit conveniently
into the format of a 35 mm camera.*

W. EUGENE SMITH

Once you can accept the universe as being something expanding into an infinite nothing which is something, wearing stripes with plaid is easy.

ALBERT EINSTEIN

Go ahead and try:

- H&M with Prada
- Vintage with a modern trend
- Plaid with stripes
- Preppy with edgy
- Masculine with feminine
- Flirty with fierce
- Funky with basic
- Leather with lace
- Sweet with vampy
- Uptown with downtown
- The precious with the not

I call it "The Kate Moss Factor." Kate Moss has this tactic down. She never looks like she is trying too hard. Something is always a bit off. Her hair is messy, her accessories don't match, her shirt is rumpled. And yet, she always looks amazing.

It's kind of painful to see girls so pristinely put together all the time. Those girls that always look like they are ready for a photo shoot do not interest me. I'm more interested in those girls who are less than perfect (perfection is overrated). They are the ones whose hair is not flawless, whose outfits are not perfectly matched, who are somehow breaking the rules. Every time I see a girl who has mastered this tactic, I smile in silent worship. They know how to live, these girls. They know how to have fun and let their hair down. They never look too perfect. These are the girls who know the most about style.

A beautiful thing is not perfect.

ANONYMOUS

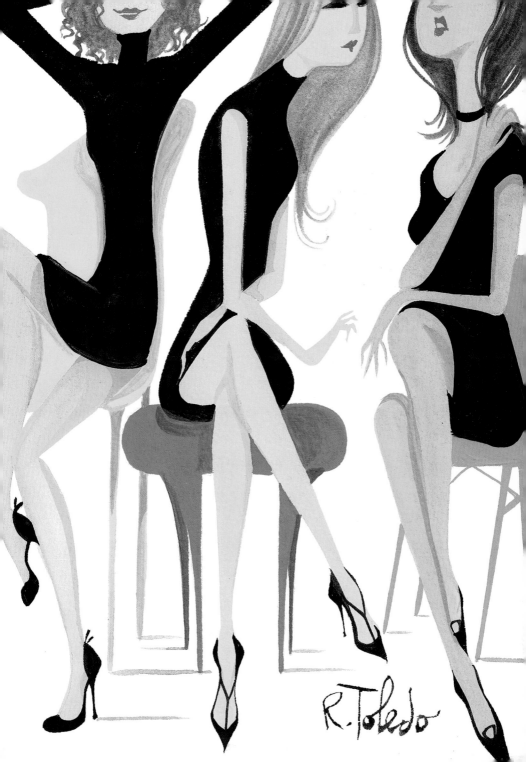

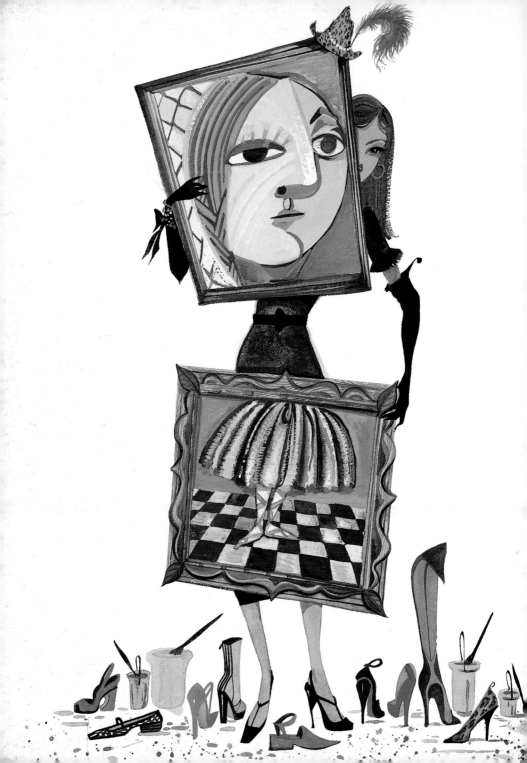

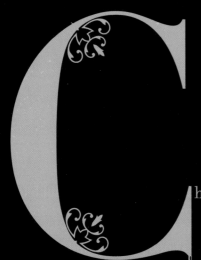

Chapter Three

INSPIRATIONS

" Those who
do not want
to imitate
anything,
produce
nothing."

SALVADOR DALÍ

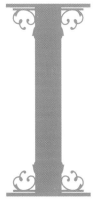

've just spent pages telling you to be your own muse, be original, and listen to your inner voice. Now I'm going to tell you to seek out other muses, to imitate, and to draw from the world around you. So maybe I'm being a bit contradictory. (I'm allowed, it's my book.) But maybe I'm not. In my mind, inspiration is an extremely personal experience and a connection with your true self. It comes from understanding a fantasy of yourself and the person you want to be. You must know this first, and then you can answer the old "What inspires you?" question. I know, it is a question usually reserved for artists and designers, musicians and actresses. But you should ask it of yourself. The stylish woman knows the answer. An artist? An actress? A rock star?

Fashion history tells us that even "the originals" imitate someone or something. They take an idea from the world, adopt an element of the image, and then make it their own. For artists and designers, inspiration knows no bounds. They find it everywhere.

John Galliano's hobo-chic look was inspired by the homeless people he saw lining the Seine when he was jogging. Vivienne Westwood adopted the fashions of the London punk rockers and made them into high fashion. Stephen Sprouse began creating his notorious graffiti collection after a day of wandering around the East Village. The designers were struck by these scenes and in some way, they connected with them. They wanted to own a piece of these worlds, so they adopted the images and adapted them to be their own.

You should look at life in much the same way. Style is about identifying who you want to be and, in order to do this, you have to seek out your inspirations. Look to the women from your childhood and from your travels. Look to art and artists, movies and actresses, music and rock stars. Find who and what you identify with, adapt them to your character . . . and then, like all great icons, live up to the part.

Anything can be a source of inspiration—nature, art, architecture, literature, travel, film, music, et cetera. Find beauty everywhere. Don't just look at things: See things. Disengage your thousand-mile stare and begin noticing details in your everyday life. Fashion, like art, music, travel, literature, and film, is one of the little gifts we get in this world. Style is a way to express your culture, your identity, your passions, and your spirit.

Have fun with it.

Style is a simple way
of saying complicated things.

JEAN COCTEAU

*Costume, hair, and makeup can
tell you instantly, or at least give you
a larger perception of, who a character is.*

COLLEEN ATWOOD

The first time you saw Uma Thurman hit that dance floor with John Travolta, tell me you didn't think her crisp, white shirt was the sexiest article of clothing ever made. (First, tell me you've seen *Pulp Fiction*.) The look isn't all that complicated: the white shirt, the black capri pants, the severe black bangs, and the bare feet. But let's be honest, it's the attitude that pulls it off. Rewind sixty seconds before the dance scene to when she tells John Travolta, "I do believe Marsellus Wallace, my husband, your boss, told you to take me out and do whatever I wanted. Now I wanna dance, I wanna win. I want that trophy, so dance good." She leads him to the dance floor, and in the next ninety seconds she forever changes our view of a simple, white shirt. Sure, the girl has her problems (she is married to a mob boss and has a bit of a cocaine habit), but she pulls off a white shirt like no other.

And during those unforgettable ten seconds in *Scarface* when Michelle Pfeiffer, in a backless aqua sheath, comes downstairs in that glass elevator, tell me you didn't envy her for just a moment.

Sure, she has her problems too (she is married to a drug lord and has a bit of a cocaine habit), but for those ten seconds she is perfection wrapped in an aqua dress and a glass elevator. And all throughout the movie, there are similar ten-second moments when you see her in her coke-head sunglasses, her slinky dresses, her perfect blond hair, and you think, *hey, being married to a drug lord isn't such a bad gig*. A pet tiger and you'd get to ride up and down your glass elevator in slinky dresses all day (or at least that's what I would do).

And for those five minutes in *The Thomas Crown Affair*, when Faye Dunaway (who doesn't have a cocaine habit, by the way) and Steve McQueen play an erotic game of chess, tell me you didn't want to learn how to play chess Faye Dunaway–style (in a pleated halter minidress, with upswept hair, fake eyelashes, and perfectly mani-cured nails). It is quite possibly the sexiest scene in cinema in which the clothes stay on. I think the dress has a lot to do with it, though her symbolic caressing of the kingpin helps too.

A minute and a half of Uma dancing, ten seconds of Michelle making an entrance, and five minutes of Faye playing chess. There are countless scenes throughout the history of film, scenes that stick in our minds and inspire us to emulate these women, or their style at least. I mean, I obviously don't suggest emulating the drug habits (remember Uma on that bathroom floor with blood spilling out her nose—very un-chic). And those relationships with wealthy criminals are never as fun as they seem (or so I've heard). But a white shirt or some coke-head sunglasses or a tapered halter dress, these things I can get a handle on.

These are the kinds of scenes that editors and designers return to again and again for inspiration and ideas. Most of what ends up on the runways and magazines starts on the big screen (Gucci based its entire fall 2006 ad campaign on Michelle Pfeiffer's Elvira character). Girls like Uma, Michelle, and Faye playing girls like Mia, Elvira, and Vicki is inspiring and it is great fun to channel a little bit of Elvira. But the trick is not to go overboard. Fictional characters can wear whatever they like; nobody is going to judge them. We must rein it in a little bit. Pick one element that you like and make it your own. Do the eighties Michelle/Elvira sunglasses, but pair them with a modern outfit. Buy a backless Faye/Vicki dress, but put on some funky jewelry and black nail polish. Wear the white Uma/Mia shirt, but don't do the black wig and capri pants unless you are going to a costume party.

WHAT TO WATCH AND WHAT TO WATCH FOR . . .

Bringing Up Baby (1938)

SETTING: New York, 1930s

SYNOPSIS: A bored society girl (Katharine Hepburn) ensnares a nerdy paleontologist (Cary Grant) and the two have a series of misadventures with her pet leopard, Baby.

STYLE: Masculine/Feminine

WATCH FOR: The movie in which Katharine debuted her signature pants, never before seen on a woman in the movies. When the studio heads insisted she wear a skirt, she strolled around the set in her underwear until they gave her pants back.

"Well, you look perfectly idiotic in those clothes."

Sabrina (1954)

SETTING: Long Island, 1950s

SYNOPSIS: After two years in Paris, Sabrina (Audrey Hepburn), the shy chauffeur's daughter, returns home as a sophisticated, stylish woman, and suddenly draws the attention of both Larrabee brothers (Humphrey Bogart and William Holden).

STYLE: Givenchy glam. This is the film that brought Hepburn and Givenchy together.

WATCH FOR: The A-line gowns and the "décolleté Sabrina," a bare-shouldered black cocktail dress with a high neckline to hide Audrey's collarbones. All the Givenchy dresses.

"Oh, but Paris isn't for changing planes, it's for changing your outlook!"

To Catch a Thief (1955)

SETTING: French Riviera, 1950s

SYNOPSIS: A former thief (Cary Grant) is suspected of a series of jewel thefts; to prove his innocence he tries to find the copycat with the help of an American heiress (Grace Kelly).

STYLE: Glistening extravagance

WATCH FOR: The jewels! Grace Kelly in that white strapless dress with an over-the-top diamond necklace. Her ball gowns, shimmering gold, blue chiffon, etc.

John: You know, back home in Oregon, we'd call you a head-strong girl.

Frances: Where in Oregon, the Rogue River?

John: Where were you born?

Frances: *In a taxi halfway between home and the hospital. I've lived in twenty-seven different towns and cities.*
John: *Was somebody chasing you?*
Frances: *Boys.*

And God Created Woman (1956)

SETTING: Saint Tropez, 1950s

SYNOPSIS: A vampy sexpot (Brigitte Bardot) loves one brother, but marries another.

STYLE: Rampant female sensuality

WATCH FOR: This is the movie that put Brigitte Bardot on the scene, and she became the instant symbol of the "sex kitten." That gingham bikini, the pouty lips, the ultimate "beach hair," and how the (near-naked) Bardot carries herself throughout the film.

Mme: *Eric, I'm worried about you.*
Eric: *Worried?*
Mme: *You are at the point of falling for her.*
Eric: *What makes you say that?*
Mme: *Whenever you look at her, you appear less intelligent.*

Funny Face (1957)

SETTING: New York and Paris, 1950s

SYNOPSIS: Jo (Audrey Hepburn), a shy bookstore clerk, is discovered by a famous fashion photographer (Fred Astaire), who takes her to Paris and makes her a top model.

STYLE: Simple, chic, casual, and then extravagant and over-the-top

Audrey Hepburn in her black capris, black turtleneck, and black flats (which made a comeback in the 2006/2007 Gap ads where Audrey is seen doing her Funny Face dance, set to AC/DC's "Back in Black." A prime example of how style persists after fifty years; there is just different music in the background). And the resplendent Givenchy gowns. The scene when Audrey descends the stairs in that stunning red Givenchy is unforgettable.

"Every girl on every page of Quality *has grace, elegance, and pizzazz. Now what's wrong with bringing out a girl who has character, spirit, and intelligence?"*

Breakfast at Tiffany's (1961)

SETTING: New York, 1960s

SYNOPSIS: Holly Golightly (Audrey Hepburn), a socialite/call girl, becomes interested in Paul (George Peppard), a struggling writer who moves into her apartment building.

STYLE: Accessorizing the LBD 101

WATCH FOR: The LBD, the oversize sunglasses, the giant pearl necklace, and the gloves. Often considered the fashion film. It solidified Audrey Hepburn as a style icon.

"I've got to do something about the way I look. I mean, a girl just can't go to Sing Sing with a green face."

Doctor Zhivago (1965)

SETTING: Russia, 1914–1917

SYNOPSIS: A Russian physician-poet (Omar Sharif) falls in love with a political activist's wife (Julie Christie) during the Bolshevik Revolution.

STYLE: Russian Revolution.

WATCH FOR: The images of Julie Christie surviving Siberia and Stalin in style largely influenced fashion in the late sixties. Mid-length officer-style coats, opulently collared and cuffed shirts, and fur on anything became popular. Lots of fur. Fur bonnets, muffs, etc. PETA's nightmare film.

"What I want to know is how we're going to stay alive this winter."

Belle de Jour (1967)

SETTING: Paris, 1960s

SYNOPSIS: Séverine (Catherine Deneuve), a beautiful young woman dissatisfied with her marriage, takes an afternoon job at a brothel.

STYLE: Perfectly timeless

WATCH FOR: Everything she wears could work today: the coats, the shift dresses, etc. Roger Vivier designed his pièce de résistance, the Pilgrim-style buckled pump, for this film. 120,000 pairs were sold immediately after the movie hit the big screen. And that same shoe is still modern today.

"For you, there is no charge."

The Thomas Crown Affair (1968)

SETTING: Geneva, 1960s

SYNOPSIS: When Thomas Crown (Steve McQueen) pulls off the perfect crime, Vicki Anderson (Faye Dunaway) is called in to investigate.

STYLE: Smart and seductive

WATCH FOR: Her nails, her (inch-long) eyelashes, her skirts, the perfectly structured, perfectly accessorized mini-suits, and that white pleated halter-neck mini in the "chess seduction scene." Every scene could make a magazine layout.

Thomas: *You play?*

Vicki: *Try me.*

Love Story (1970)

SETTING: Cambridge and New York, 1970s

SYNOPSIS: After graduation, a rich Harvard law jock (Ryan O'Neal) marries a poor Radcliffe music student (Ali MacGraw).

STYLE: Preppy collegiate.

WATCH FOR: The coats, cozy sweaters, and the notable hat and scarf sets—Ali MacGraw's knit stocking cap became an instant craze.

Jenny: *You're gonna flunk out if you don't study.*

Oliver: *I am studying.*

Jenny: *Bullshit. You're looking at my legs.*

Oliver: *You know, Jenny, you're not that great-looking.*

Jenny: *I know. But can I help it if you think so?*

The Great Gatsby (1974)

SETTING: Long Island, Summer 1922

SYNOPSIS: A film adaptation of F. Scott Fitzgerald's classic, in which Jay Gatsby (Robert Redford) falls for the flighty Daisy Buchanan (Mia Farrow).

STYLE: WASP American style and the return of the twenties flapper

WATCH FOR: Mia Farrow's cream and white flapper dresses, her long beads, wide-brim hats, the pin-curl bob. Redford's Ralph Lauren–designed three-piece suits, driving caps, and gloves.

"I've never seen such beautiful shirts before."

Mahogany (1975)

SETTING: Chicago, 1970s

SYNOPSIS: Tracy (Diana Ross) tries to leave the ghetto and become a fashion designer and a top model.

STYLE: Outlandishly retro. Diana Ross designed some of the costumes herself. Marc Jacobs based his fall 2007 collection on this film.

WATCH FOR: The retro designs, the color, and the glitter. The ombre evening dress. White pantsuits. Seventies turtlenecks. The hair.

"Hair has always been important."

Annie Hall (1977)

SETTING: New York, 1970s

SYNOPSIS: A neurotic comedian (Woody Allen) falls in love with the neurotic and ditzy Annie Hall (Diane Keaton).

STYLE: Androgynous chic. The masculine/feminine. Tutorial in how to wear our boyfriend's clothes.

WATCH FOR: Keaton's hat, man's tie, shirts, waistcoats, and wide-leg pants.

"Well la-de-da!"

American Gigolo (1980)

SETTING: Beverly Hills, 1980s

SYNOPSIS: Julian Kaye (Richard Gere) is the highest-paid male prostitute in LA (naturally). He falls in love with the wife of a local politician (Lauren Hutton) and is framed for the murder of one of his clients.

STYLE: American chic at its best. This is the film that put Armani on the style map. Lauren Hutton epitomizes effortless American sportswear. And Richard Gere becomes the first Hollywood actor to appear full-frontal nude on screen (just FYI).

"I made you! I taught you everything you know! How to dress, table manners, how to move, how to make love ..."

Scarface (1983)

SETTING: Miami, 1980

SYNOPSIS: Tony Montana (Al Pacino), a young Cuban refugee, is drawn into Miami's underworld of crime, cocaine, and Elvira Hancock (Michelle Pfeiffer).

STYLE: The look of unadulterated debauchery. Long before the rebirth of South Beach, there was the glamazonian beauty of Elvira. Gucci's spring/summer 2006 advertising campaign was based on Elvira's look.

WATCH FOR: The slinky, shiny dresses, the huge coke-head sunglasses, the blond hair.

"Say hello to my little friend!"

Pulp Fiction (1994)

SETTING: Los Angeles, early 1990s

SYNOPSIS: The lives of two mob hit men, a boxer, a gangster's wife (Uma Thurman), and a pair of diner bandits intertwine.

STYLE: Hip simplicity. Uma Thurman in the dancing scene is amazing. Her capri pants, her crisp white shirt with the black bra underneath, her severe bangs, and black hair. Amazing.

WATCH FOR: The black capri pants, the white shirt, and the hair.

"All right, everybody be cool, this is a robbery."

In the Mood for Love (2000):

SETTING: Hong Kong, 1962

SYNOPSIS: Chow Mo-wan (Tony Leung) and Su Li-zhen (Maggie Cheung) form a close friendship when they discover their spouses are each having an affair.

STYLE: Everything in this movie is styled to perfection.

WATCH FOR: The color of her dresses, the 1950s heels, the quiet sexiness of the fit. A prime example of the international woman.

"You notice things if you pay attention."

When Debbie Harry ripped her tights and hiked up her skirt, American girls followed. When the Beatles went hippie psychedelic on the world, the world went hippie psychedelic too. And when Madonna rocked that Gaultier bustier in her Blonde Ambition tour, well, we noticed. Music and personal style are so closely linked that no musician can escape them. Not even a scruffy rocker from Seattle (though Lord knows he tried).

In the early nineties, when Kurt Cobain came onto the scene in his flannels, thermals, and oversize cardigans, American teenagers copied the look, scouring thrift shops for old flannel shirts. In his Perry Ellis spring 1993 collection, Marc Jacobs did the same. He explained the moment of inspiration, saying, "I remember being in Berlin the year the wall came down, and I was in some bar, and 'Smells Like Teen Spirit' was on the radio." When he came back to New York, he found a two-dollar flannel shirt on St. Marks Place (very Nirvana) and sent it off to Italy to have the plaid pattern made into silk (very un-Nirvana). Soon he was sending silk flannels, satin Birkenstocks, and duchesse satin Converse down the runway. I will never forget those Birkenstocks. I had my first internship at Perry Ellis during the spring 1993 season and I spent a good amount of my time running satin Birkenstocks around New York for editors to use in their photo shoots. Nobody returned them, so I also spent a good amount of the internship saying, "I promise you, there are no more," and watching how Nirvana's look became a high-end rage at the same time it was a high school craze.

What follows is a list of rock stars and musicians that have

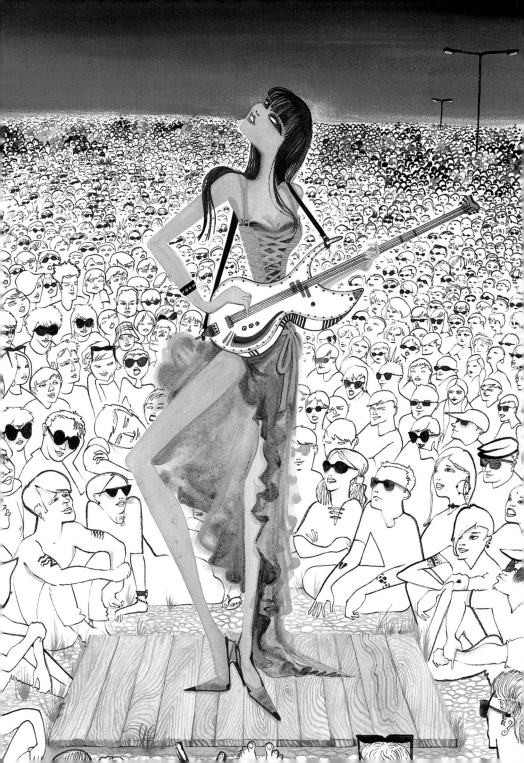

influenced style and fashion on a large scale. They are icons who designers and editors pull from again and again to create their collections and their magazine spreads.

Musicians with Style: The Set List

- Diana Ross and The Supremes
- Cher
- Janis Joplin
- Patti Smith
- Debbie Harry
- The Rolling Stones
- The Sex Pistols
- Tina Turner
- Madonna
- Kurt Cobain

DIANA ROSS AND THE SUPREMES

"With the Supremes I made so much money so fast all I wanted to do was buy clothes."

—DIANA ROSS

They were all glamour and 1950s sophistication with their gowns, wigs, detailed makeup, white gloves, pearls, and piled hair. They used sequins, gold lamé, feathers, and chiffon. They wore tight skirts, jackets, sleeveless dresses, and even Chanel-inspired two-piece suits. Everything they wore put an emphasis on their curves and their femininity, their signature look being glamorous evening gowns with gloves and high heels.

CHER

"I've always taken risks, and never worried what the world might really think of me. Until you're ready to look foolish, you'll never have the possibility of being great."

She introduced California cool to the world. She made long, straight hair popular and introduced tight bell-bottomed jeans and the exposed midriff. She wore seventies flower-print dresses with white go-go boots. Her clothes always had a flash of something: color, feathers, sequins, glitter.

JANIS JOPLIN

"Don't compromise yourself. You are all you've got."

Joplin haunted the thrift stores and friends' closets looking for unique pieces. She customized her clothes with embroidery and beading. She wore cowboy boots with long boho skirts, threw leather and tie-dye into the mix, and piled on accessories, because she liked the jangle of jewelry. She was rock's first female star and she invented her own style, becoming a master of the mix.

PATTI SMITH

"There weren't a whole lot of female images that I could grab on to. So a lot of my influences were male. As far as I'm concerned, being any gender is a drag."

She could easily be mistaken for a boy, and that was the point. She dressed just like a teenage boy would. She wore tight rubber pants, showing off her drainpipe legs. She wore loose undershirts, bringing attention to her long, thin arms. Or she would layer: cardigans over T-shirts, topped off with a waistcoat. Or she would mix lengths: a long masculine shirt with a short masculine vest and a riding jacket. She often wore combat boots and always kept her hair messy. Patti Smith blurred the lines between men's and women's fashion in the 1970s, and the rest of the world caught on a decade later.

DEBBIE HARRY
"I am the party."

She was the first punk-rock princess. She wore short black shorts, strategically ripped tights, acid-green dresses, tube tops, and had peroxide-blond hair. She loved to break the rules, wearing short, short skirts with her curvy figure; flaunting her inventive do-it-yourself clothes made out of tacky Woolworth fabrics; buying her sunglasses at the dime store. It was her blend of sex and strength that made her a style icon and a symbol of the eighties. Later, singers like Madonna, Courtney Love, and Gwen Stefani would all attribute their styles to her.

THE ROLLING STONES
"Please allow me to introduce myself, I'm a man of wealth and taste."

They were rebellious and raunchy. They sang about honky-tonk women and not getting any satisfaction. They wore tight corduroy pants, velvet jackets, silk shirts, ruffled shirts, and exaggerated black-and-white makeup, and they grew their hair long. "They look like boys whom any self-respecting mum would lock in the bathroom," wrote the *Daily Mail*. Their rebellious and revolutionary clothing reflected their hard-edge image and will always be the example that designers return to when they want to achieve a rock-star vibe. Because nobody knows how to rock out like the Stones . . . and I'm not sure anybody ever will.

THE SEX PISTOLS

"I'm not chic. I could never be chic."

—SID VICIOUS

They shredded their jeans, shaved their heads (or donned Day-Glo Mohawks), put spikes on their leather jackets, tore their stockings, pierced their bodies, and ripped and then safety-pinned their clothes. They were the leaders of punk rock. They commanded an audience, perpetuated a movement, and forever changed the fabric of pop culture . . . with shredded jeans and safety pins and screams of "anarchy in the UK" (all while being outfitted by Vivienne Westwood).

TINA TURNER

"Physical strength in a woman—that's what I am."

The miniskirt, lipstick, and spiked, wild hair. She is one of rock's most glamorous icons. She has always been known for her daring and edgy outfits (and her amazing legs). Her popularity and her overpowering stage presence earned her the moniker "Queen of Rock 'n Roll." Her short skirts and big hair have secured her a spot in fashion immortality.

MADONNA

"Better to live one year as a tiger, than a hundred as a sheep."

"Gonna dress you up in my love / All over, all over. . ."

There is nothing daring or controversial that Madonna has not embraced or created. She introduced us to yards of lace, teased-out hair, leather, spandex, and bright colors. Madonna was the eighties and we worshiped at her altar (with yearbook and wedding pictures to prove it). And then, just as everybody jumped on board, she reinvented herself, in true Madonna fashion.

Her career evolved with carefully planned stylistic phases. There was her lacy underwear, big hair, and black jewelry phase; the sultry Marilyn Monroe phase; the *Evita* phase; the Japanese geisha; the uninhibited sex goddess in Gaultier (with Blonde Ambition). She has always been, and continues to be, on the cutting edge. She is the queen of reinventing herself. Nobody will forget the Gaultier bustier, the men's suits, the leather gowns, the girl-on-girl kissing, the Kabbalah strings . . .

KURT COBAIN

"I feel stupid and contagious. . ."

In the early nineties, Kurt Cobain emerged out of suburban Seattle in a ratty flannel, a beat-up pair of Converse All-Stars, and a dirty cardigan. Soon his look was strolling down the runways of New York, Paris, and Milan, thanks to Marc Jacobs in his infamous "grunge collection," and celebrities were buying the items at hundreds of dollars a pop. The youth of America achieved the look for much less. They went into thrift stores for the clothes; they grew their hair long and purposely neglected to wash or comb it. It was an era of antifashion, but in an odd way, it was the only decade that can be so identified by a singular fashion trend.

"The world is a book, and those who do not travel read only a page."

ST. AUGUSTINE

Style and Travel

I was smart enough to come along fashionably late, a full ten years after my older sister. By the time she was in boarding school, my parents were ready to globe-trot, so I trotted along too. My father was right, there was always time to get caught up on long division (though I'm not sure I ever have), but there is nothing like walking through the halls of the Louvre or watching an Italian woman move through the streets of Rome. These are the informal lessons a girl doesn't soon forget. Wherever we went, I would notice how differently women dressed in each country. I would also watch as my mother picked up the styles, buying the necklaces and dresses and bringing them back to Colombia. These women—the women of the world and my mother—showed me how the best sources of inspiration are often found outside of your area code. It doesn't matter where you go; it's what you bring home.

SOUTH AMERICA

"I don't go out without makeup. I'm a woman, you know."

—SHAKIRA

South America is the land of the beauty queen. These women put a lot of time and effort into the way they present themselves (humidity be damned). I don't think I once saw the women in my house leave without putting lipstick on. It just doesn't happen. There is a strong focus on femininity and standards of personal grooming that the South American woman adheres to every single day. The standards are not only a matter of presentation, but a matter of moral fiber. There is a notion, passed down from generation to generation, that your physical presentation reflects the person you are on the inside. Through everyday pageantry, there is an aura of effortless chic and a display of correctness inside and out that never lets up.

EUROPE

"Sex appeal is fifty percent what you've got and fifty percent what people think you've got."

—SOPHIA LOREN

In Europe, it is all about tradition. European women are the consummate embracers and masters of style; they have made fashion an art form. For these women, style is never created; it simply is. And it has meaning. Take the Hermès bag, for example. The French woman carries hers because it is an heirloom, not because it is an "it bag." And she will wear a certain scarf because her grandmother wore it. For this woman, the power of tradition shapes her entire process of elegance.

ASIA

"You mustn't be eaten by the kimono. You must eat the kimono."

—HANAYAGI GENSHU

Throughout Asia, style is laced with ritual and culture. The geisha, for example, with her unremitting attention to luxuriant, theatrical beauty, has cultivated a sense of feminine mystery for centuries. At the other end of the spectrum, you will also see in the streets of Tokyo the progressive zeal of the Japanese youth. They are the masters of urban chic, with their fingers on the pulse of modernity. In both cases, style is underscored by authentic devotion to detail, artfulness, and grace.

INDIA

"Pink is the navy blue of India."

—DIANA VREELAND

On a daily basis, the women in India are ensconced in extreme color, sparkle, and texture. They wear endlessly ornate, gold-and-enamel jewels quite unabashedly, with silken saris of every hue. The important events of their lives are usually punctuated by a ritualized approach to the kind of beauty that is laden with custom and tradition. At an Indian wedding, the bride, dripping with handcrafted jewelry and shrouded in exquisite veils, is as much an example of sumptuous embellishment and personal beautification as she is a woman on the way to her future.

AFRICA

"We have to approve of ourselves before anyone else will. Women need to celebrate their God-given beauty instead of always trying to be something else."

—IMAN

For women in Africa, ornamentation has always been paramount to style, and their perspective is reminiscent of queens and goddesses. Elaborate head wraps, luminous colors, organic textures, and jewels of all kinds characterize the impacting power-beauty of the African woman. For obvious reasons, these women have had to reclaim their style throughout the centuries, forging an even stronger sense of pride and alliance to these roots.

THE UNITED STATES

"She was an American girl, raised on promises."

—TOM PETTY

The United States is the place where a phenomenon like the blue jean was born, and where women were liberated from the austere demands of old-world dressing codes. It is a country with distinct styles throughout the regions. In the Southwest, you'll find turquoise jewelry and cowboy boots. In LA, women adore boho dresses and peasant tops. In New York, you can find just about anything. In America, the promises of possibility and inspirations are limitless.

Anything that might catch your eye is worth the trek, but you do not have to travel far. If you cannot get away, go to the ethnic shops in your neighborhood. But wherever you go, be it Tokyo or the local Indian store, this is the time to buy with drama. Bring back something fantastic. Pull out all the stops. Humidity be damned, forget about modesty, leave the trends behind, and have a little fun.

*One should either be a work of art
or wear a work of art.*

OSCAR WILDE

Style and Art

The influences here are legion. They are found in The Met and the Louvre, but they are also found on graffitied walls and old flea-market prints. Every designer has been influenced by art, and art has been influenced by style. There is an intense amount of cross-over between the two. Paul Poiret, the famed designer from the early 1900s, is credited as the first to champion the designer/artist connection. "I have always liked painters," he said. "It seems to me that we are in the same trade and that they are my colleagues." And Poiret mentored Elsa Schiaparelli, the designer who is widely regarded as the first to really meld the two worlds. From there on out, every designer has sought out artistic inspiration. There are countless notable marriages of art and style; I am going to give you my favorite three:

SALVADOR DALÍ AND ELSA SCHIAPARELLI

In 1936, Salvador Dalí created his famous Lobster Telephone, a functioning phone with a lobster carcass for the receiver. The connection was perfectly clear to him: "I never understand why, when I ask for a grilled lobster, I am never served a cooked telephone." In 1937, the Lobster Telephone inspired Elsa Schiaparelli to create her famous Lobster Dress, a virginal white dress with a red sash and a two-foot red lobster printed on the front. She had Dalí, her good friend, design the fabric. The connection was perfectly clear to her; for Elsa Schiaparelli, there was nothing that could not be used for inspiration. She made connections between her clothing and the world around her as no one had before. And she was the first to design entire collections around a theme (and everyone followed suit). She would use African iconography or sailors' tattoos or musical instruments or butterflies or pagan imagery. The woman knew how to be inspired. She knew how to imitate an image, but also to claim it as her own. This is a woman we can learn from. She let everything influence her style. Imitate her.

YVES SAINT LAURENT AND PIET MONDRIAN

This is one of those moments when the crossover is very recognizable and clear cut. In the twenties and thirties,

Dutch painter Piet Mondrian designed positional, graphic paintings. The compositions were gridded with thick black lines and basic primary colors. YSL took this design idea and fit it to the female form, creating his famed Mondrian collection. The dress became a phenomenon in the 1960s; the collection has remained one of the most recognizable art/fashion intersections. But YSL's artistic inspirations go much deeper than Mondrian. He explained, "Naturally, there was Mondrian, who, in 1965, was the first I dared to approach and whose rigor captivated me. But there was also Matisse, Braque, Picasso, Bonnard, and Léger. And how could I possibly have resisted Pop Art, which was the expression of my youth? How could I have overlooked my dear friend Andy Warhol? And how could I not have borrowed from van Gogh—his irises, his sunflowers, his wonderful colors?" His attitude and approach to art and fashion have become a standard that other designers constantly look to for inspiration.

MARC JACOBS AND STEPHEN SPROUSE AND TAKASHI MURAKAMI

In the late nineties, Louis Vuitton hired Marc Jacobs as fashion director, and Jacobs soon began to seek out artists to bring a new vision to the company. In 2001, he collaborated with graffiti artist/designer Stephen Sprouse to design limited edition Vuitton bags with graffiti scrawled over the LV monogram pattern. They only created a very limited number, and Sprouse's friends began to buy regular LV bags and asked him to put graffiti on them.

In 2003, Jacobs met with Takashi Murakami, and the two masterminded the Monogram Multicolore design, which featured the original LV monograms in thirty-three different colors on either white or black backgrounds, instead of the traditional gold monograms on a brown background. Murakami also created the Cherry Blossom pattern for the company, stamping smiling cartoon faces and pink and yellow flowers atop the original monogram canvas.

Jacobs's collaborations with both Sprouse and Murakami clearly display the "fashion as art" and "art as fashion" mentality, which the fashion world has embraced wholeheartedly.

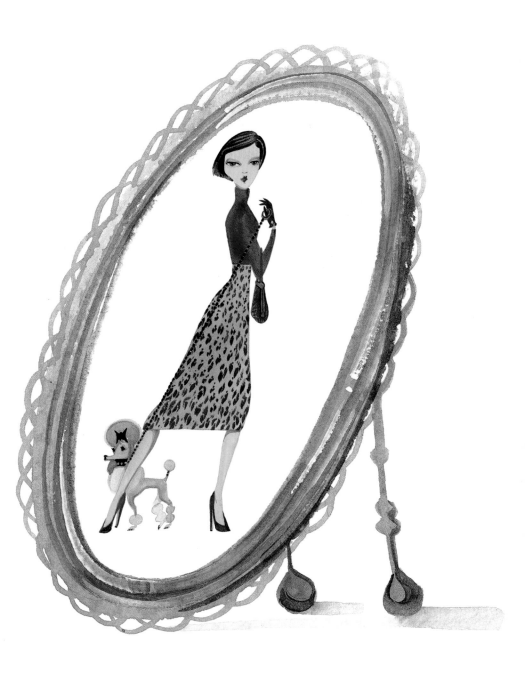

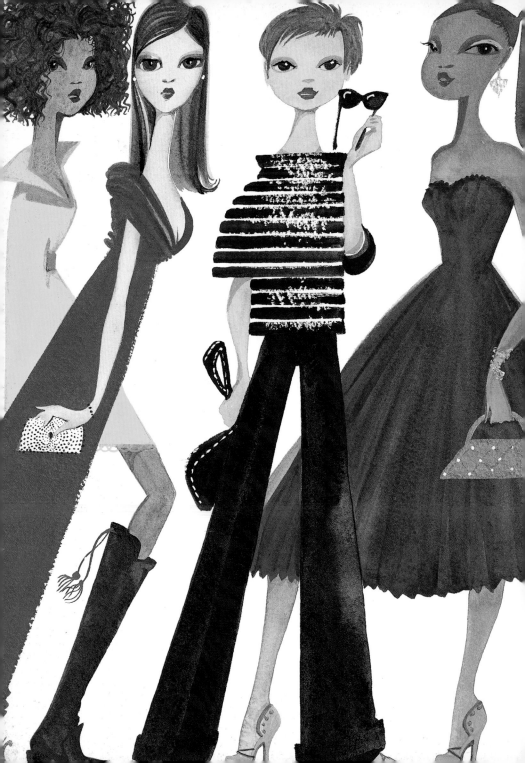

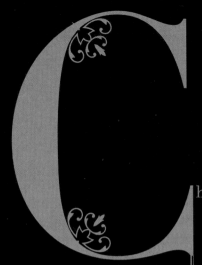

Chapter Four

WHAT TO WEAR WHEN. . .

"I wear my sort of clothes to save me the trouble of deciding which clothes to wear."

KATHARINE HEPBURN

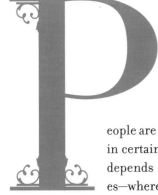**P**eople are always asking me what they should wear in certain situations. There is no one answer. It depends on so many different circumstances—where you are going, what you are doing, the weather, the season, the time of day, and on and on.

But since you've asked, here are a few of my suggestions. . . .

Know, first, who you are;
and then adorn yourself accordingly.

EPICTETUS

HOW TO DRESS WHEN THERE IS A DRESS CODE

Always read invitations carefully. I have been a victim of this. Walking into a black-tie affair in dressy casual attire is not fun. You want to show up to the party and make a statement. The statement should be "Wow," not "Whoops."

Black tie

In the evening, you are to become the butterfly. This is the time to carry out the fantasy of who you want to be. Wear bold colors, wear fabulous jewelry, wear anything that helps you make a statement and an entrance. For a black-tie affair, men are required to wear a tuxedo and women are expected to be in a long dress or a cocktail dress. But this is the time to come out of your cocoon. Don't be just another woman in a long black gown; there will be plenty of those to spare.

Some tricky variations: white tie (ball gowns), formal (same as black tie), creative black tie (this means there is a theme; always be wary of themes and make sure you don't look costumey).

Cocktail attire

This means a short dress. Have a lot of fun here. Pull out that fabulous short dress, your killer high heels, your funkier jewelry. Big cocktail rings are made for this dress code.

Some tricky variations: black tie optional, informal, semi-formal (all mean practically the same thing).

Dressy casual

This means pants are okay but no jeans. Fun tops are great, but don't do a T-shirt.

Some tricky variations: smart casual (same as dressy casual), festive casual (another theme dress code—be careful), business casual (no low-cut tops).

Casual

It means anything goes. But not for you. Someone is extending an invitation to you, so make the effort. You have a lot of freedom. Have fun with it.

HOW TO DRESS ON A PLANE

Do not wear a sweatsuit. Not even an expensive one. Because let me tell you, if there is a girl in a sweatsuit and a girl in a cashmere sweater and there is the possibility of an upgrade, cashmere beats sweatsuit every time. The way you present yourself matters: The nicer you look, the nicer you will be treated. The smile gets more than the frown.

On a flight from New York to LA, I was traveling with an actress who got on the plane in perfect attire, perfect hair, full-on makeup, and sunglasses. When we got off that plane in LA, not a hair was out of place. She looked as if she had been beamed there in a spaceship (damn her). I am not saying we all need to look this perfect (I'm sure I was a mess in comparison), but we should meet halfway between perfection and sweatpants.

Never go on trips with anyone you do not love.

ERNEST HEMINGWAY

Switch into the sweatpants on the plane if you want, but for the airport, put on nice pants or jeans instead. And then layer, layer, layer. A cashmere cardigan and a cashmere scarf are necessities on an airplane. Bring a light trench or jacket and a nice, handsome tote, and a pair of sunglasses (which can be worn the whole flight if you don't want to put on makeup). As for the shoes, wear flats. This is one of the few times when you should not wear high heels. It is not all that fun (or glamorous) to run for your flight in high heels.

HOW TO DRESS ON A FIRST DATE

It should be about mystery. It's about making them wonder. A slow reveal is more intriguing than a full reveal. Focus on the fabrics and not exposing too much skin. Silk, cashmere, angora, or anything tactile work well. This is the time to pull out your favorite lingerie (not for him, for you!), because even if the date is a disaster, at least you will feel happy. Be at ease, be superfeminine, and roll with the awkward pauses.

Is not the most erotic part of the body wherever the clothing affords a glimpse?

ROLAND BARTHES

HOW TO DRESS WHEN MEETING THE BOYFRIEND'S PARENTS AND/OR POTENTIAL IN-LAWS

Okay, no pressure here, but his mother is never going to forget what you have on when you first meet her. Don't ask him, he knows nothing. He's just going to say, "I'm sure whatever you wear will be fine. My mother is going to love you." Ha. We all know that the mother comes to that table full of judgment and doubt. You have to come to that table full of poise and style.

You never get a second chance
to make a first impression.

EVERYONE'S MOTHER

Clearly this is not the time to wear a low-cut shirt or your fishnet stockings or your S&M boots. She's probably not going to like that. This is also not the time to show lingerie. This is the time to be a little conservative. Knee-length skirts are good, miniskirts are not. Wide-leg trousers, yes. Shredded jeans, no. Cardigans work, cleavage does not. That's all common sense. But do not make the mistake of completely changing your style to impress them. You have to show them who you are, just not *all* of who you are. Wear classic, nonrevealing clothing, but make sure your bag, or your necklace, or your watch reveals a bit of your style.

And, this has nothing to do with what you wear, but don't be one of those fake, smiley girls. Don't forget it's not just *your* mother with a pitch-perfect bullshit detector. His mother has one, too. They are built in during pregnancy. The fathers? They're a little easier to fool.

HOW TO DRESS ON A JOB INTERVIEW

The low-cut shirt, fishnet stockings, and S&M boots probably won't work here either. Again, you are going to have to be a little conservative, but in most cases you don't have to wear a suit anymore. You do have to consider where you are applying. A pencil skirt with a button-down shirt and nice heels will take you almost anywhere. If it's a fashion magazine or an art studio, you can throw in a trendier top. It's about mixing and matching. At a law firm or a finance office, you'll have to toe the line a bit more. If you do want to go the suit route, make sure it is a very well-tailored suit—it has to look amazing. Invest your money here.

As a general guideline: Choose a conservative base and then put on a piece of personal jewelry, something that says you are alive and not a robot in a suit.

No one has ever had an idea in a dress suit.

FREDERICK G. BANTING

If you're wearing lingerie that makes you feel
glamorous, you're halfway there to turning heads.

ELLE MACPHERSON

I once saw one of the most influential women in fashion wearing one of her standard amazing outfits: a great jacket with a great pair of jeans. But when she turned around, I was horrified. Panty lines! Granny panties! Who in the twenty-first century does not own a thong? That day she fell from grace just a little bit (or maybe a lot). You have to check your backside before leaving. No panty lines or thongs showing!

Pay as much attention to your lingerie as you do to the rest of your outfit. Use it to your advantage. Don't shy away from playing with color, layering, and trying very feminine, vintage finds. Explore garters, corsets, etc. It's like opening Pandora's box. Just do not use a bra as a top. It's ridiculous and not at all provocative. And, really, everyone knows you are wearing a bra. But a leopard print or lacy bra that shows just a little bit can be incredibly seductive (just don't show too much of it).

You should have the basic colors for those times when only a classic bra will do, but be wary of nude bras. It can look like you have a prosthetic breast (not a good look). It can work quite well when absolutely needed, but it's not the most seductive shade.

Yes, most of the time, only you are going to know what you have on underneath your clothes, but wear great lingerie anyway. A little optimism never hurt anyone.

HOW TO DRESS ELEGANTLY

Your shoes, bag, and coat will reveal your hand right away. Spend your money here. A simple, timeless design for these three items is best. A classic high heel, a quilted leather bag (think Chanel), and a knee- or mid-calf-length coat all work well.

Isn't elegance forgetting what one is wearing?

YVES SAINT LAURENT

Keep it simple and understated. For the pants and top, choose a rich color—camel, brown, ivory, or black—and wear them tone on tone. For example, an incredible pair of ivory pants and a luxe ivory turtleneck equals elegance. Head-to-toe black, brown, and camel work the same way. (It doesn't matter how much the pants and the turtleneck cost, looking elegant is not about the money.) Then add a great coat and choose some lasting jewelry: a charm bracelet, bangles, hoops, a cocktail ring, turquoise, coral, or pearls.

I think I have monogamy. I caught it from you.

SAMANTHA, *SEX AND THE CITY*

First of all, avoid being a bridesmaid. It answers your question of "what to wear" right away, but at a ghastly cost. Second, do not wear white. For some reason, people get very touchy about that. Especially the mother of the bride. Most important, you have to consider where the wedding is. Again, read that invitation carefully. If it's a night-time wedding in the city, dress as you would for black tie. If it's a daytime wedding on an island, a flirty sundress. If it's an afternoon wedding at a country club, wear a simple shirt and top, accessorize, and prepare yourself for whale-print belts. If it's a 3 a.m. wedding in Vegas, anything goes.

HOW TO DRESS FOR A SUMMER WEEKEND

Look at that shot of Jackie in Hyannis in her jeans and T-shirt and perfect summer accessories. And look at Brigitte Bardot in *And God Created Woman*, showing off a gingham bikini and tousled beach hair. These women knew how to do summer.

Summer weekends are for letting your hair down, naps in the

sun, margaritas on the back deck. Jeans and T-shirts are key here. Sundresses and tank tops and just one great bathing suit are essential too. Keep everything simple and then punctuate your outfit with all of those summer accessories that seem like they were made for lazy Sundays in July—the flat sandals, the sun hat, the L.L. Bean tote.

The best-dressed woman is one whose clothes wouldn't look too strange in the country.

HARDY AMIES

Keep it cool and casual. Nobody wants to go to the beach with a woman in high heels and a leather Prada bag. Everyone wants to go spend the weekend with Jackie O. or Brigitte Bardot.

HOW TO DRESS FOR WINTER

Has a woman who knew she was well-dressed ever caught a cold?

FRIEDRICH NIETZSCHE

Get a great coat. It is what everyone is going to see you in, so you have to make sure it's amazing. Find one that has a bit of flair—a bright color, a distinct pattern, a standout collar, oversize buttons—anything that's going to make you stick out in the sea of black and brown. I am a fan of black and brown in the winter, but not for the coat. A woman in a plain black coat rarely makes an entrance. A woman in a black mink? Yes. A woman in a red trench? Yes. A woman in a black peacoat? Eh. Everything else can be black, if you want. Black pants, black shoes, black turtleneck. Just have that splash of color or pattern in your coat and you're golden.

The colors for winter are pretty standard: black, brown, gray, camel. You can't go wrong there. But definitely dare to wear winter white and ivory. There is nothing more chic than a woman in winter white. The dry cleaning bill is worth it. Also worth it: anything cashmere (which most certainly can be found for cheap) or alpaca (which most certainly cannot). And, PETA be damned, I am a huge fan of fur. It will keep you warm and you will look instantly luxe. If you can't afford the coat, buy the hat. If you can't afford the hat, ask your older relatives for their castoffs and take them to a tailor to be redesigned. Nothing is better to rework than an old fur coat. And nothing will make you feel more glamorous in the depths of December.

HOW TO DRESS WHEN PREGNANT

Wear jewelry. Lots of jewelry. Make the guy buy it for you—he got you into this. He can help you style your way through. Instruct him to find you bangles, earrings, fun necklaces. Anything to take the focus off the belly. It doesn't have to be anything fancy or exorbitantly

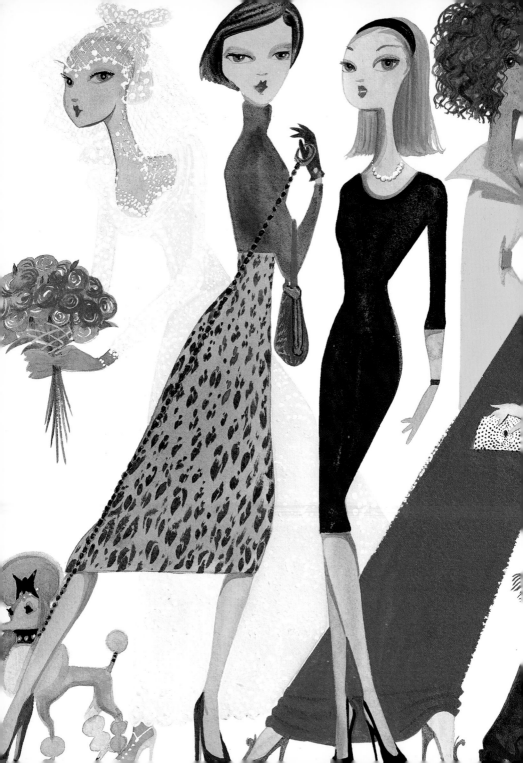

expensive (though don't tell him that—if he wants to spend, who are you to stop him?).

Whatever you do, don't try to hide your belly by wearing big, baggy clothes. It will just make you look bigger, and really, that's not what you need right now. What you need is a few fitted cashmere sweaters (in the winter) or cotton T-shirts (in the summer) that will hug your body perfectly and not make you look like a beach ball. To further stave off the beach-ball silhouette, you'll also need a good pair of maternity jeans. Make sure they are comfortable, snug on your hips and thighs, and flare out a bit at the ankles to balance out the belly. Do not buy maternity jeans that are tapered at the ankle. You are going to look like a Weeble (and Weebles wobble . . .). Don't be afraid to spend money on any of these items. Comfort takes precedence over credit card debt during these glorious (right) nine months.

Sadly, you're probably going to have to hang up the high heels for a few months. I wake up and go to bed in heels, and even I couldn't pull it off for nine months. Ballet flats are your friend here. They are extremely comfortable and flexible enough to stretch out as your feet start to expand (very attractive).

Have I made this sound fun enough for you? There are plus sides to the whole pregnancy gig. Your hair gets thicker. Your boobs get bigger. You are going to "glow" (or people are going to tell you that, anyway). You can send people out to get you cheesecake in a snowstorm and they won't say a word.

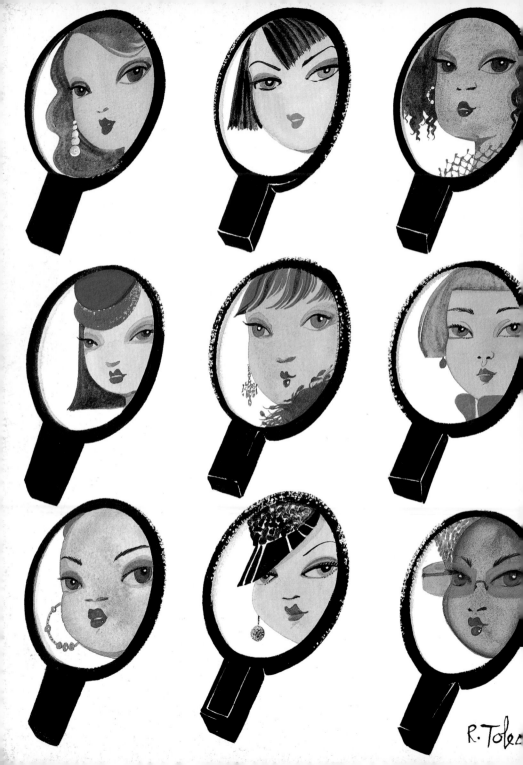

R. Tole

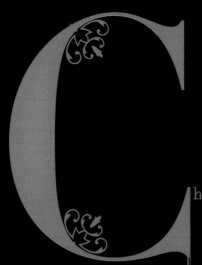

Chapter Five

INSIDER TIPS AND TRICKS

"Don't give a woman advice; one should never give a woman anything she can't wear in the morning."

OSCAR WILDE

DIANE VON FURSTENBERG,
on inspiration and confidence

Q: What was your inspiration for the wrap dress?

A: I was really very young, in my early twenties. I worked in an Italian factory and I loved printed jersey. It started as a little wrap top like a ballerina would wear, and then one day I just had this idea to make it into a dress. It is the most traditional dress, like a kimono, but it was revolutionary because it was made out of jersey and it was tight to the body.

Q: What is your secret to staying young?

A: I love life and I live it fully.

Q: What is your favorite item of clothing?

A: Whatever I am wearing at the moment. There is that moment in the morning when you put on the right thing and it somehow feels like the right thing.

Q: The secret to style?

A: You have to figure out where you are going and what you have to do and then just go for it.

ZAC POSEN,
on self-assurance and making an entrance

Q: What do you find stylish in a woman?

A: Each woman has her own allure. I like humor, opinion, and self-assurance.

Q: Who are some of the most stylish women you know?

A: They know who they are.

Q: Expert tips on how to dress for a party?

A: Dress the part you want to play.

Q: How to dress to make an entrance?

A: The same way you make an exit: with aplomb, shoulders back, and a withheld secret.

TORY BURCH,
on the timeless versus the trendy

Q: What is your secret to blending timeless and trendy styles?

A: If I wear a trendy shoe or piece of jewelry, I keep the rest of my outfit simple and stick to classic pieces with clean lines.

Q: How do you recognize if something is a trend versus something that is going to last?

A: A trend is usually something that lasts for only a season or two. Classic pieces like a crisp white shirt or a timeless khaki trench will never go out of style.

Q: What is your favorite source of style inspiration?

A: Vintage photographs—I am inspired when I look at pictures of chic women from the sixties and seventies. Women like

Jane Birkin and Catherine Deneuve had such an innate sense of style.

Q: What do you find most stylish in a woman?

A: The confidence to wear what looks good on you regardless of trends. Women who dress to play up their assets and hide their flaws always look polished and pulled together.

Q: Who is the most stylish woman you know?

A: My mother. I remember watching her get ready for an evening out when I was little and thinking she was the most glamorous and chic woman I had ever seen. I still feel the same way when I look at her today.

CAMERON SILVER,
on buying and wearing vintage

Q: What are the secrets to buying vintage?

A: Quality and modernity. Vintage is not about dressing retro, but rather about incorporating pieces from the past to give you a thoroughly modern look that is distinctive and showcases your unique personal style. But junky vintage in poor condition will not fit the bill. Try to look for things that have been well cared for and are high quality.

Q: Is vintage for every woman?

A: There is vintage for every woman. Okay, I am not saying everyone can wear late-eighties Sant'Angelo stretch gauze, but accessories are a great way to incorporate vintage and they're one size fits all. Sometimes a more mature woman feels she can't wear a vintage piece of clothing, but I disagree. It's about dressing appropriately for your age and size, and vintage is part of an equation for all women with a desire to be distinctive.

Q: What is the best vintage item a woman can buy?

A: A great vintage Hermès bag, be it a Kelly, a Constance, a Birkin, or something more rare and out of production. It is the epitome of quality and taste and will be passed on to future generations.

Q: What do you find most stylish in a woman?

A: I am drawn to women with a unique sense of style. I appreciate those who dress authentically eccentric as well as those who dress classic and iconic. I think it's the individuality that shows through a woman's choices that create a stylish woman.

Q: Who is the most stylish woman you know?

A: Nina Garcia! Hey, that's a loaded question since I must be very diplomatic about this. But I adore Chloë Sevigny's style, as well as my friend Liz Goldwyn's. Tatiana Sorokko and Susan Casden . . . but there are too many to name just four!

RALPH LAUREN, on breaking the rules

"I have always believed that breaking rules is what makes clothes interesting. It is what I've done in different ways for my entire career. I love mixing fabrics and shapes in unexpected ways—the classic with the modern, the rugged with the elegant. There are no limits, as long as it's done with a certain taste level."

GILLES MENDEL, on fur

Q: How do you pick your first fur?

A: Your first fur should be the coat you always dreamed about, a fantasy object that makes you feel special every time you slip it on, and, of course, if it also happens to keep you warm, that is an extra plus.

Q: Is there anything fur does not go with?

A: Fur or a touch of fur will complement any look. It adds a touch of glamour and luxury; it can do wonders as a pick-me-up for a plain little black dress.

Q: What is the biggest mistake women make when wearing fur?

A: Treating it as something you can only wear on a special occasion. Now we treat fur like an extraordinary fabric that can easily become part of a lifestyle. Fur is no longer just your grandmother's mink that came out on special occasions. Fur is a modern luxury item like cashmere that can be enjoyed at every price by everyone.

Q: What do you find eternally stylish?

A: The perfectly cut tuxedo or a classic trench coat.

Q: Who are the most stylish women you know?

A: I still love Jane Birkin and Kate Moss.

FRANCISCO COSTA,
on minimalism with allure

Q: What is it about a white shirt that is so appealing?

A: A white shirt always looks crisp and sexy. It's a fashion staple.

Q: What is your favorite article of clothing on a woman?

A: The skirt is the most feminine article of clothing on a woman and can dictate the whole silhouette.

Q: How does a woman dress with minimalism without looking boring?

A: One should always refer to the proportions to update the silhouette—the same old dress can look exciting in a new length.

Q: What is the best lesson you have learned from Brazilian women?

A: Brazilian women know how to let the sensuality speak for itself

MARGHERITA MISSONI,
on dressing in prints and the fun part of fashion

Q: What is your secret to dressing in prints?

A: As with anything, you just have to feel comfortable in them. If you don't, don't even try. If you are uncomfortable in bold colors or anything drastic, it's not going to look good.

Q: Can you mix prints?

A: Yes, definitely. It depends what you are going for. If you are going for a hippy seventies look, you are going to mix prints.

If you go for gypsy or boho, you mix. I don't see prints as constricting. I see prints as pieces that you can mix just as you mix different shapes and volumes.

Q: Can you wear prints to a wedding?

A: Yes, I often do. I think you wouldn't wear anything too bold or too bright, just as you wouldn't wear anything white. You never upstage the bride. Don't go for something that is too much. Lighter-color prints are good.

Q: Who or what has influenced your style the most?

A: You can be influenced by everything you see and everywhere you go. I was lucky to grow up in a situation and environment where there were a lot of people with a peculiar sense of style, so I always had a bigger, broader view of what could have been. Nothing was strict and precise, which is the fun part of fashion.

Q: Who is one of the most stylish women you know?

A: Carine Roitfeld.

Q: What are the secrets to European women's style?

A: Be yourself. In America, women are more worried about wearing the "right thing," fitting in, and following the "right trend." In Europe, they follow their instincts more, which leads to an individual sense of style.

ELLE MACPHERSON,
on lingerie, personal style, and attitude

Q: What are your insider tips on buying lingerie? Wearing lingerie?

A: Make sure it fits properly. Most women do not know their real bra size. Experiment with color (most colors don't actually show under white).

Q: What is the biggest mistake women make when buying/wearing lingerie?

A: Not buying matching bra and knickers. In bathing suits, less is more. In lingerie, more is more!!! (Two knickers for every bra, even better.) Try medium g-string or boy-leg, depending on the mood and clothes.

Q: What are your tips for achieving a personal style?

A: Find a personal style by not following fashion trends. I have worn jeans and a white T-shirt with knee-high/cowboy/motorcycle boots, ballet flats, and a cashmere jumper for twenty-five years. The shape of the jeans changes and that's about it. I believe in comfort and consistency. There is something disquieting about clothing schizophrenia.

Q: Who has been your biggest source of style inspiration?

A: I think the seventies were a period that affected me as a teenager (my mum was a teenager too, practically). We lived in flared jeans and waistcoats and platforms. Surfing and rock and roll are the sorts of lifestyles that have affected my choice in clothes.

Q: What do you find stylish in a woman?

A: A woman is stylish no matter what she wears if she is comfortable in her skin. I love when a woman is uncontrived and simple with a sense of inner strength. She could be naked or in a ball gown and her attitude does not change.

Q: Who is the most stylish woman you know?

A: I believe there are so many women who have their own "stylish style." Angelina Jolie always looks effortlessly beautiful. Talitha Getty had fabulous eclectic taste. Julie Christie's style (her hair and makeup) is unbeatable. Audrey Hepburn is magnetic and palatable in *Breakfast at Tiffany's* (everything she put on looked amazing). Cate Blanchett has a face and poise and inner wisdom and dynasty. My friend Elizabeth Saltzman always looks amazing.

Q: What is your favorite article of clothing?

A: A white Vince T-shirt.

ISABEL TOLEDO,
on strong shapes

Q: What is the secret to buying and wearing a strong shape?

A: The secret to wearing strong shapes is BODY LANGUAGE—a woman has to be comfortable in her own skin to make strong shapes work for her. Once you know yourself and understand how to use your body language, clothes with shape

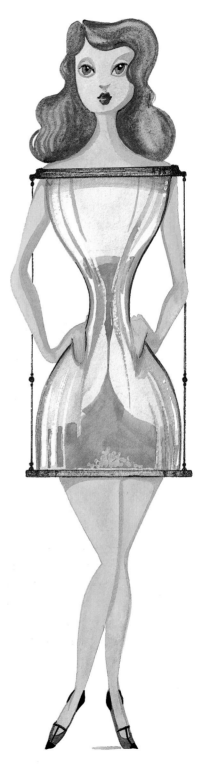

can enhance your graphic presence and help to project your own personal style.

Q: What is your secret to mixing the practical with the fantastical?

A: This is the essence of style for me. How you mix opposites and rearrange realities to get at a deeper truth. I love the practical and build everything around it first. Fantastical just happens when you are open to it and can evaporate just as quickly. It has been my experience that from the fantastical, often the practical is born.

Q: What is one item of clothing every woman should have in her closet?

A: Underwear!!! For me, a wonderful wardrobe of exquisite underclothes is the ultimate luxury. It is what you first put on, and no matter what your look is, there is nothing that can elevate your mood as much as what you have on underneath it all. Different undergarments for different types of clothes are essential in order to make a look work for you.

Q: What do you find eternally stylish?

A: Good grooming is the one thing that is a permanently stylish element. When you are perfectly groomed, you can conquer the world . . . even in a pair of old jeans and a T-shirt!

Q: Who are some of the most stylish women you know?

A: I adore the classic generations' sense of ageless style. Maria Felix, Louise Bourgeois, Iris Apfel, Anna Piaggi, Louise Nevelson, Frida Kahlo—they have all shown us that an independent and confident sense of yourself is what it is all about. Diana Vreeland, who I had the fortune to intern with at the Costume Institute at the Met, had that gift all through her life—the joy of living and dressing up or down for any challenge. We had the same shoe size and she would insist on trying on my picks that I found on Canal Street. That curiosity and enthusiasm is a real gift and the reward of a fertile mind and an open spirit—that is what fuels fashion!

REED KRAKOFF,
on handbags and summer weekends

Q: What is the one bag every woman should have?

A: A big classic tote that goes with everything—the iconic American bag.

Q: What is your favorite accessory for a woman to wear?

A: A handbag, for obvious reasons. Seriously, anything that brings out her true personality.

Q: What should a woman wear on a summer weekend?

A: Something casual and chic. Nothing too forced, as if to look like she tried too hard. After all, it is the weekend.

Q: On a first date?

A: Nothing too sexy or revealing. You may want to leave something to the imagination.

Q: What is the sign of a stylish woman?

A: Unique, confident, timeless.

Q: Who is the most stylish woman you know?

A: My wife Delphine—effortlessly chic at all times. Dressed up or casual—day or evening.

MICHAEL KORS,
on cashmere, crocodile, and comfort

Q: What one item should all women own?

A: Brown crocodile stiletto pumps.

Q: What should a woman wear on a plane?

A A black cashmere turtleneck and white jeans and huge sunglasses.

Q: Which fabrics work best for seasonless dressing?

A: Matte jersey. It is sexy and comfortable and is the best to travel in.

Q: What are the hallmarks of modern sportswear?

A: The combination of comfort, sex appeal, and luxury.

Q: What do you find incredibly stylish?

A: Women who look unstudied, yet elegant at the same time.

Q: Who is the most stylish woman you know?

A: Gwyneth Paltrow.

IMAN, on confidence and smiles

Q: How to be confident?

A: Be comfortable in your own skin. Don't follow trends. Only wear what looks good on you, but update it. Rock whatever you wear and smile, honey, smile!

Q: What do you find stylish in a woman?

A: Confidence in her choices regardless of what others think, and a sense of irony.

Q: What is your favorite piece of clothing?

A: Either a white shirt or black turtleneck—both modern, classic, elegant, casual, and timeless.

Q: Who or what has inspired your style?

A: My mom. She dressed without apology.

FRIDA GIANNINI,
on reinvention and reinterpretation

Q: What is the key to reinventing old pieces?

A: I love vintage clothes, and I love scouring different markets for great treasures, which serve as a source of inspiration. I like to compare the lines, details, and colors of what I find with what I am interested in now. The references and reinterpretations satisfy a curiosity, but they should never be literal. I draw a lot of inspiration from the Gucci archives, specifically iconic elements such as the horsebit, crest, and bamboo. Updating an iconic print by putting it on a fresh silhouette perfectly marries tradition with modern innovation.

Q: What should a woman keep in mind when mixing textiles?

A: For me, mixing contradictory elements makes the most interesting and successful combination. I love a style from the 1970s paired with a very modern shoe silhouette, or a vintage tote bag with bamboo handle paired with this season's dress shape.

Q: What or who is your main source of inspiration?

A: Inspiration can be found anywhere and everywhere. I find it from young men and women on the street or from movies,

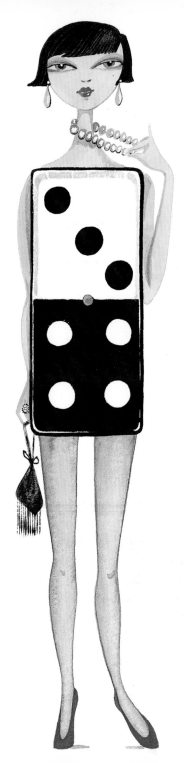

from fabrics, from music, from art, from architecture, and from literature. I take inspiration from different fashion eras and different fashion icons.

Q: Tips on wearing accessories?

A: Accessories are an integral part of a collection and are used to frame every look. Whether it is a bag or shoe, pin or cuff bracelet, accessories complete every image. There are no rules with accessories, and one should experiment with shapes and sizes of bags, boots, or even jewelry.

JOHN GALLIANO,
on not giving a damn

Q: Is too much really never enough?

A: Too much imagination? Too much fun? Too much excitement? Too much adventure? NO WAY! Enough is never enough and when you are tired of the routine you have to go seek adventure so that you never get enough—feed your mind, body, and soul, and live life in a technicolor of imagination.

Q: What one item should be in every woman's closet?

A: A lover—that something seductive to get them there!

Q: How have different cultures affected your designs?

A: Styles, cultures, women from around the world are like different timbres of music—there is so much to dance to. You should never stand still.

Q: What do you find eternally stylish?

A: The great Dodie Rosenkrans—she has the eye, the style, and the imagination that makes her the Peggy Guggenheim of the fashion world, and I am honored to be a part of her collection!

Q: Who is the most stylish woman you know?

A: Kate Moss—always has been—always will be. She dresses for herself, for her mood, and that is what makes her WOW!

Q: What is glamour today?

A: Confidence, independence, not giving a damn, and going for it—glamour is luxury, quality, knowing your stuff and indulging your desires—in fashion, life and living.

SANTIAGO GONZALEZ,
on precious skins

Q: What should a woman look for when buying a croc bag? Or any precious skin item?

A: The most important thing is to look at the way the skin is placed on the product. It should be center cut, meaning the belly of the skin should be centered on the bag or wallet, making the scale completely balanced on each side. And the less seams it has the better. Fewer seams indicate a much finer product.

Q: What other textiles can a woman mix with precious skins?

A: Precious skins are the ultimate luxury accessory. They go with any textile, color, and style. The beauty of skin is that every product is unique. Each product is a collaboration with nature. The scales and patterns are never going to be the same, so every bag becomes unique, with its own personality.

Q: What is the biggest mistake woman make when buying/ wearing precious skins?

A: People think that because it's a luxury item, they should buy it in black or brown. But accessories are meant to accessorize! It's all about the experience. They are supposed to make you feel good. Black and brown are always basics, but turquoise or red might bring a more joyful experience.

Q: What do you find timelessly stylish?

A: A great design should not only be timeless, but should also be universal. It should appeal not only to every age, but also to every time period and style. The same product should be applicable and valid to all generations. These are the hallmarks of a "classic."

Q: Who is the most stylish woman you know?

A: Style is something very personal. All women are stylish as long as they are original and authentic.

CAROLINA HERRERA,
on elegance and Latin American style

Q: What is your secret to elegance?

A: For me, less is more.

Q: You always make something as simple as a white shirt look chic, what is your secret?

A: It is not only about the white shirt, it is the way you wear it and how you mix it for the right occasions.

Q: What has been your biggest source of style inspiration?

A: Life, in general, is great inspiration. You can take things from all around you and put them into the right context. A lunch with friends, laughter, books, art, gardens, colors, my memory; anything can inspire me.

Q: What is the key to Latin American style?

A: The Latin American style is very seductive. It is not only what you wear, but the way you move, dance, laugh, talk, that makes it so special.

Q: What do you find stylish in a woman?

A: Attitude and confidence is very important.

Q: Who is the most stylish woman you know?

A: Daphne Niarchos.

OSCAR DE LA RENTA,
on glamour and good taste

Q: What is the secret of glamour?

A: Discipline.

Q: Why do your clothes appeal to women of so many ages?

A: They appeal to women of so many ages because true women of today are ageless.

Q: What are the hallmarks of good taste?

A: It is all in the eye of the beholder.

Q: How do you dress a woman for a black tie event? A cocktail party?

A: In what she feels will be most alluring and will project her sense of individuality.

ROBERTO CAVALLI

Q: What is the key to wearing animal prints?

A: Look for your natural inner animal magnetism. Be confident and have fun with fashion.

Q: Advice for women on wearing color?

A: Color is positivity. Always choose a color according to the mood of the day. A colorful dress can have amazing powers.

Q: What is the secret to Italian style?

A: Enjoy life and live every minute to its fullest.

Q: What do you find eternally stylish?

A: A woman who takes care of her appearance at every age.

Q: Who is the most stylish woman you know?

A: Every woman who feels confident with her body.

DONATELLA VERSACE,
on sex appeal and that certain something special

Q: What is the key to looking sexy at any age?

A: Fashion, glamour, sensuality—these are not qualities reserved only for the young. The more life experience a woman has, the more confident and alluring she becomes. The

Versace woman may be a sassy twenty-two-year-old or she may well be a glamorous forty-five-year-old. What these women have in common is the knowledge that strength and confidence are among their most powerful qualities; sexy is a state of mind.

Q: Tips for how to dress on a plane?

A: Thirty years ago, people wore their best suits and outfits to travel—now, track suits are the norm. Dressing up gave these occasions a certain importance. It made these little things more glamorous and I miss that. You can be comfortable without ever compromising glamour.

Q: What is one article of clothing every woman should have?

A: I think the most valuable item a woman should have is not actually a piece of clothing; it is an accessory. Women these days are so busy that they do not have time to change their clothes every other minute, or to completely revamp their closets with all of the latest trends—that's why accessories have become so important. With just a quick switch of a handbag or a pair of shoes, you can instantly change your look and mood. High heels are probably my biggest obsession; I love the glamour and sex appeal of that perfect pair.

Q: What do you find stylish in a woman?

A: Without a doubt, the most stylish asset that any woman can have is confidence. Versace is a lifestyle that personifies many different interests and passions. It is nearly impossible to create and fulfill a path that is truly yours if you do not believe in yourself. The Versace woman is not only confident in her tastes and style, but also steadfast in her beliefs. The Versace woman has a way about her. You may not be able

to put your finger on it, or even describe it, but you will recognize this woman the moment she walks into a room.

Q: Who are some of the most stylish women you know?

A: The most stylish women I know are those that have a certain
something special. With strength and innate femininity,
these women can rule a red carpet, have a relaxing brunch
with friends, or even revel in a spontaneous spring shower—
all without batting an eye. Strong, confident, and ever-so-
alluring, she has a magnetic charm that challenges the status
quo. Madonna, Demi Moore, and Halle Berry are among the
most stylish women I know.

CHRISTOPHER BAILEY,
on trench coats and other staples

Q: What items, besides a trench coat, should every woman have
in her closet?

A:

· The perfect, crisp, white man's shirt (including lots of
Jermyn Street–type striped shirts)
· A great, well-cut, sexy pair of jeans
· An iconic Burberry Manor bag
· Lots of cashmere polo shirts in all colors
· A tailored sartorial jacket

Q: What are your tips for mixing classic style with street style?

A: A relaxed attitude, good tailoring, handmade English shoes,
and a smile.

Q: What is the best way to wear a trench in the summer? Winter?

A: A trench can be worn over an evening dress, a pair of jeans, or a jogging pant, there are no parameters with the classic.

Q: What do you find amazingly stylish in a woman?

A: Inner peace.

Q: Who is the most stylish woman you know?

A: I love Charlotte Rampling, although I have not met her.

RACHEL ZOE,
on drama and the red carpet

Q: What is one piece of advice you give all of your clients?

A: There is never an excuse not to be glamorous.

Q: What is the key to looking Hollywood chic?

A: Not to look like you tried too hard, but to put in that effort when you are off camera.

Q: What are the most important elements for being red carpet ready?

A: Always have proper undergarments and great posture. Bad posture ruins any look.

Q: What is the best thing to wear to a black tie?

A: Something other than black. If it is black, it has to be dramatic. And wear more costumey accessories. Big and bold. Not dainty. I like drama.

Q: A cocktail party?

A: Always do a short or knee-length dress. No gowns. The key here is to find that middle ground between overdressing and underdressing, which is attained by choosing rich fabrics, great jewelry, great heels, and a red lip.

Q: A first date?

A: First, you have to find out what you are doing and where you are going (i.e. if you are going to a movie, you are not going to wear a dress, unless it's a sundress). The key is to look cool and comfortable. You don't want to be fidgeting and fussing in your clothes. And you also don't want to look like it took you ten hours to get ready. Again, be comfortable.

Q: What do you find eternally stylish?

A: Those classics, like a Birkin bag or a Chanel bag. And those trends that do not date, like a red lip and fabulous lashes.

Q: Who is the most stylish woman you know?

A: Carine Roitfeld.

VICTOIRE DE CASTELLANE,
on jewels...lots of jewels

Q: What is the difference between how French women wear jewelry and how American women wear jewelry?

A: I think French women wear what they love and do not hesitate to mix different styles of jewelry in a more bohemian way. They are not afraid of wearing multiple pieces at the same time, layering them as a means of expressing their own style. Americans respond more to wearing statement pieces individually, like an amazing ring or necklace that stands out on its own. Whether it is large or small, bold, or delicate,

Americans approach wearing fine jewelry in a classic way.

Q: What is the one piece of jewelry every woman should have?

A: A huge, colorful ring.

Q: What is the best thing to wear to a black tie?

A: It depends on each individual. It can be either a fantastic pair of earrings or an enormous ring.

Q: On a first date?

A: It is better to wear a piece of jewelry that makes you feel beautiful. And then the gentleman knows what kind of jewels you love and what to offer you for the second date!

Q: Where do you find inspiration for your designs? For your personal style?

A: For my designs, my inspiration comes from everywhere: from fashion, the street, the movies, exhibitions, and even fairy tales. As for my personal style, my feminine shapes are my inspirations! I know skirts and dresses are for me. After that, I mix everything I like.

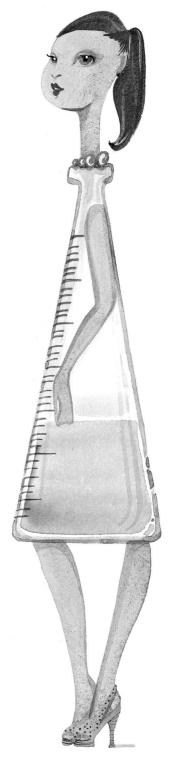

Q: What do you find most stylish?

A: I like feminine clothing, especially high heels. I love the style of women from the movies of the 50s and 70s; their mood was so carefree. They were holding cigarettes in hands adorned with unbelievable rings and amazing bracelets on their wrists. I also like women who talk and gesture in such a way that makes their jewelry seem alive.

Q: The most stylish woman you know?

A: It is hard to mention one person in particular since today there are so many women who possess a unique sense of style. A woman who mixes her jewels as she wants is what I consider to be the most interesting. I like women such as Helena Rubenstein and Barbara Hutton—my grandmother's best friend—who in their time wore hundreds of jewels together and looked very extravagant.

CHRISTIAN LOUBOUTIN,
on shoes and red soles

Q: What should a woman look for or avoid when shoe shopping?

A: Depending on the ankle, avoid the ankle strap. If you have a great leg, then great, but the ankle strap can cut off the leg instead of elongating.

Q: What is the one shoe every woman should own?

A: A classic black pump with a four-inch straight heel.

Q: Why the red sole?

A: It's a green light for men.

HEIDI KLUM, on bras, undies, and muu-muus

Q: What is the key to dressing stylishly sexy?

A: I think the key to dressing sexy is to not try overly hard. It's
much sexier when it all appears a bit effortless. You can tell
when someone looks uncomfortable in their skin—clothes
that don't fit properly or don't fit the wearer's personality
definitely don't help, so I think it's important to wear something you feel gorgeous in.

Q: Advice for women on buying and wearing lingerie?

A: I have lots and lots of lingerie. I'm a Victoria's Secret "An-
gel," so you can bet that my lingerie drawers are full of cute
undies and bras! I personally like seamless and small lingerie. On an ordinary day, I think it's fun to wear sexy lingerie,
even if you're running around in your sweats. And one trick
I tell guys who are shopping for gifts for their wives or girl-
friends is to buy a small size . . . better than to buy a big size
and have the girl be like "Hey!" . . . she can always return it!

Q: What is the secret to dressing well when pregnant?

A: I don't think there is a secret to pregnancy dressing. I hardly bought any maternity wear ... instead, I just wore a lot of
loose, comfortable jersey and cotton dresses, long tanks and
tees, and bought jeans a few sizes too large for me normally
and wore them low. I'm not a fan of wearing muu-muus. I
think it's better to show off your belly—it's beautiful and
natural!

Q: What do you find eternally stylish?

A: I think that non-fashion victims are eternally stylish—
people who just have their own style, their own way of

putting themselves together with a unique flair, who aren't slaves to trends and know what looks good on them!

Q: Who is the most stylish woman you know?

A: I personally think my mom is super stylish. She likes to look youthful and modern, and when we go shopping together, sometimes she's the one who gets the "hipper" stuff!

VERA WANG, on weddings

Q: What is the most common style mistake a bride makes?

A: I think the worst mistake a bride can make is not to be recognizable. The essence of who she is sometimes gets lost after everyone gets hold of her. Be true to your own style. If you normally dress conservatively, your wedding is not the time to try something risqué. The most important thing is to wear something that makes you feel beautiful.

Q: How can bridesmaids be stylish?

A: The same rules that apply to the bride apply to her attendants as well. Do not make any extreme or unusual beauty statements. Jewelry should always be minimal, and natural makeup looks best. A pale color can be subtle and more romantic for a summer wedding, while dark colors look great in winter. Low backs or slightly décolleté necklines can be sexy and highly appropriate during summer months; obvious cleavage, however, is never tasteful.

Q: What is your advice for guests when dressing for a wedding?

A: Regarding issues of wedding attire, everyone must defer without exception to the bride. The hour, season, and venue should dictate the choice.

Q: What do you find incredibly stylish in a woman?

A: Women have to be true to themselves. You should adhere to your personal style, no matter what the situation. A woman is never sexier than when she is comfortable in her clothes.

DOMENICO DOLCE & STEFANO GABBANA,
on confidence and style

Q: What is the key to choosing a perfect little black dress?

A: A woman needs to know her body type, how to show off certain areas and hide others . . . to enhance her figure and embrace her curves. The little black dress is a must-have.

Q: What is the secret to Sicilian style?

A: The secret to Sicilian style is always dressing confident and sexy.

Q: What do you find eternally stylish?

A: Besides the little black dress and stiletto pumps, definitely one's inner style. A woman that embraces both herself and her surroundings . . . she is polished, elegant and sophisticated.

Q: Who is the most stylish woman you know?

A: There is no particular woman, it is the attitude of a woman—how she carries herself, whether on the beach, walking down the street or at a red carpet premiere. She should exude confidence, charisma; the beauty and style will happen on their own.

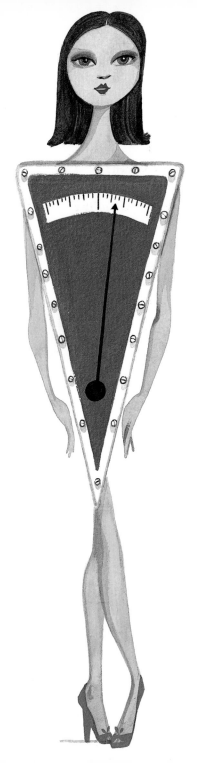

Q: What constitutes elegance in a woman?

A: One could devote an entire book to answering this question. Alternatively one can respond to it in the briefest possible terms: It is the result of a natural equilibrium between simplicity, looking after oneself, and intelligence. All this generates the poise and special attitude we call elegance. It is a quality which, contrary to popular belief, does not require deep pockets.

Q: Who is the most elegant woman you know?

A: She is one whom I got to know through books and magazines: the magical Coco Chanel, who invented everything and wore it herself, painting her own accurate self-portrait through her fashion. Truly she was the most elegant woman I have known, and the most elegant of the twentieth century. If we are looking for someone from our own time, then I would choose Cate Blanchett, a strong woman who knows what she wants. She has a natural and very modern beauty; her film star glamour enhances the most lavish dresses. She has a magnificent presence, and her character serves to underline her humanity.

Q: Which accessory should every woman aspire to own?

A: One that matches her own personality, that in some way speaks on her behalf, something that is not strictly utilitarian but is an essential reflection of her taste and pleasures. A long, eye-catching necklace, perhaps, in crystals and semi-precious stones, or a pair of earrings to frame the face. But in my opinion, nothing is as indispensable as a minaudière made of unusual and precious materials; almost a piece of jewelry rather than a handbag.

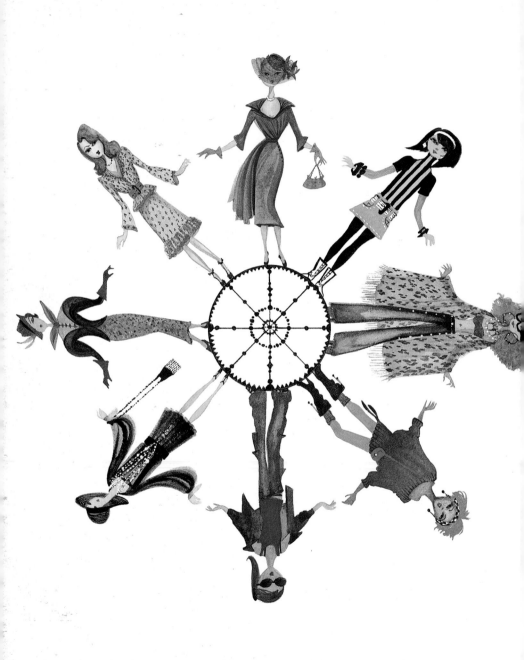

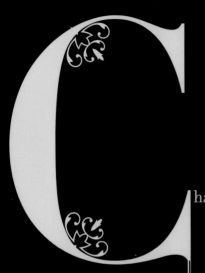

Chapter Six

FASHION CLIFF'S NOTES,
DECADE BY DECADE

"In order to be irreplaceable, one must always be different."

COCO CHANEL

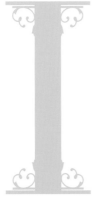

I f you find yourself at a table full of fashionistas and everyone is dropping names (which hardly ever happens), this should help you get by....

1920s

THE TRENDS TO KNOW: the flapper, bobbed hair, higher hemlines, lower waistlines

THE NAMES TO KNOW:

- GABRIELLE "COCO" CHANEL—jersey-knit dresses, two-tone shoes, the LBD
- JEAN LANVIN—complex trimmings, embroideries, and beaded decorations in light, clear, floral colors
- JEAN PATOU—introduced sportswear for women, knitted swimwear, the tennis skirt
- PAUL POIRET—his heyday was pre-1920 (circa 1909–1914), when he helped liberate us from the corset and introduced the world to female pantaloons; he designed through the twenties

1930s

THE TRENDS TO KNOW: return to femininity and glamour, backless dresses, nylon hosiery

THE NAMES TO KNOW:

- MADELEINE VIONNET—flowing, feminine clothes; created the cowl neck and the halter top
- ELSA SCHIAPARELLI—first to use art in her clothing; also used zippers, shoulder pads, buttons, bright colors (her signature "shocking pink")
- MADAME GRÈS—revolutionary in her intricate draperies and impeccable cuts

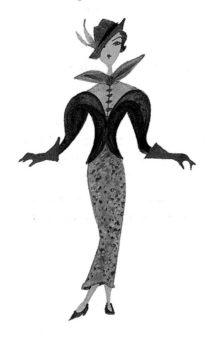

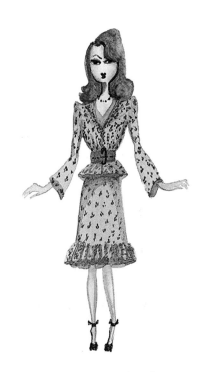

1940s

THE TRENDS TO KNOW: day dresses, blouses with bow detailing, military looks

THE NAMES TO KNOW:

- CHRISTIAN DIOR—reestablishes Paris as fashion center, revives haute couture, reintroduces glamour with "The New Look" (tight waist, stiff petticoats, billowing skirt), signifies the end of the war
- BONNIE CASHIN—made boots a major fashion accessory
- CLAIRE MCCARDELL—first American sportswear concept for women

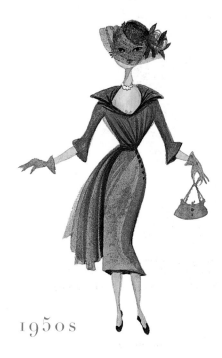

1950s

THE TRENDS TO KNOW: high heels, pencil skirt, shape and volume

THE NAMES TO KNOW:

- CRISTÓBAL BALENCIAGA—brought us balloon dresses, tunic dresses, chemise dresses, and the empire line
- GIVENCHY—first "marriage" of a designer and a movie star (Audrey Hepburn), made the little black dress famous, introduced separates
- CHANEL—returns, bucks "The New Look," introduces the famous braided suit with gold chains, costume jewelry, monogrammed buttons, quilted bags on chains

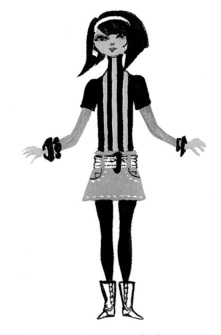

1960s

THE TRENDS TO KNOW: "mod," fun revolutionary clothes, short skirts, psychedelic prints, wild colors, go-go boots, dresses made of vinyl, paper, cellophane, metal, covered in mirrors, baby-doll dresses

THE NAMES TO KNOW:

- PIERRE CARDIN—the first ready-to-wear lines
- MARY QUANT—champions the youth movement, introduces miniskirt, hot pants, launches Twiggy
- YVES SAINT LAURENT—opens fashion house, makes safari chic
- EMILIO PUCCI—psychedelic prints, first clothes for the jet-set
- PACO RABANNE—uses metal, paper, plastic in his designs
- ANDRÉ COURRÈGES—father of the mini, uses cutouts, peepholes, sheer tops
- RUDI GERNREICH—worked with vinyl and plastic, launched the "monokini" (topless bikini)

1970s

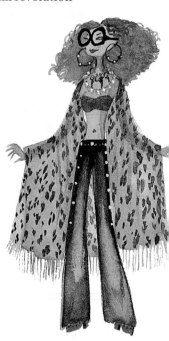

THE TRENDS TO KNOW: disco, ethnic trend, bell bottoms, miniskirt, platform shoe

THE NAMES TO KNOW:

- VIVIENNE WESTWOOD—mother of the punk revolution
- SONIA RYKIEL—makes knitwear fashionable, uses dark blacks, rhinestones, long boa-like scarves, crocheted hats
- GEOFFREY BEENE—debuted geometry and fashion
- BILL BLASS—puts American style on the map
- ELIO FIORUCCI—glam rock style, bright rubber boots, fake fur, pop art jackets
- CALVIN KLEIN—defines a brand by advertising
- RALPH LAUREN—introduces the first lifestyle brand
- NORMA KAMALI—revolutionizes swimwear with her "pull bikini"
- ANNE KLEIN—brings us American women's sportswear

1980s

THE TRENDS TO KNOW: a decade of color, power suits, and the Japanese invasion

THE NAMES TO KNOW:

- AZZEDINE ALAÏA—sexy and seductive designs with an emphasis on the figure
- JAPANESE INVASION—Yohji Yamamoto and Rei Kawakubo of Comme des Garçons and Issey Miyake all brought Eastern fashion to the world stage
- DONNA KARAN—brought a feminine approach to the ready-to-wear
- TOMMY HILFIGER—made preppy Americana chic, later adopted by hip-hop
- BILL BLASS—he took American sportswear to its highest level; adored by businesswomen and executives' wives.
- PERRY ELLIS—a new wave of American sportswear, used color and natural fibers, elegant variations on the basics
- PRADA—Miuccia Prada, niece of company's founder, began to produce ready-to-wear fashion that mastered "the mix"
- CHRISTIAN LACROIX—creates the pouf skirt
- MANOLO BLAHNIK—makes the shoe as important as the dress
- JEAN PAUL GAULTIER—took lingerie details and made them fashion (Madonna and the corset)

1990s

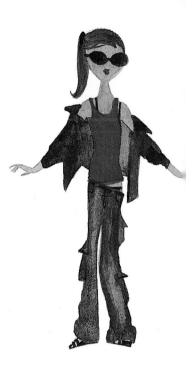

THE TRENDS TO KNOW: minimalism, simplicity, and grunge

THE NAMES TO KNOW:

- MARC JACOBS—brought grunge to the catwalk
- TOM FORD, FOR GUCCI—showed the world how to sell sexy
- GIANNI VERSACE—daringly sexy with a lifestyle to match
- DOLCE & GABBANA—superfeminine clothes for the modern-day Sophia Loren
- ROBERTO CAVALLI—rich hippy designs; used animal prints, feathers, and leather
- THE ANTWERP SIX—six designers, all graduates of the Royal Academy of Fine Arts in Antwerp, brought us the vision of contrasting elements, including: Ann Demeulemeester (mixing of unusual fabrics), Dries Van Noten (mixing classic designs with a highly personalized aspect), Walter Van Beirendonck (mixing violently divergent colors)

THE TRENDS TO KNOW: the superbrand is born, music moguls as designers, and the handbag becomes all-important

THE NAMES TO KNOW:

- ALBER ELBAZ, FOR LANVIN—brings back femininity and romance with silk, pleated dresses, satin ribbons
- CHLOÉ—brings back girly style, vintage-inspired tops, and sexy trousers
- JOHN GALLIANO—master of the dramatic
- KARL LAGERFELD, FOR CHANEL—the reinvention of all of Coco Chanel's classic staples, and created the cult of Coco LV—the birth of the designer handbag
- OSCAR DE LA RENTA—dresses all first ladies (regardless of political party)
- ZAC POSEN—clothes that make an entrance
- CHRISTIAN LOUBOUTIN—Red-soled shoe, darling of A-listers everywhere

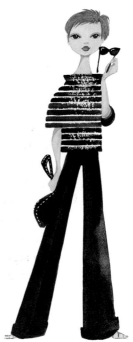

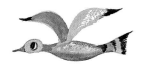

If a girl looks swell when she meets you,
who gives a damn if she's late? Nobody.

THE CATCHER IN THE RYE

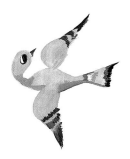

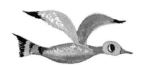
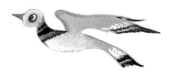

A Few Thoughts. . .

I HAVE SPENT A GOOD MANY SEASONS watching fashion trends come and go, style myths created and dismantled, hemlines rise and fall. The one solid piece of advice I have to offer is: don't take it all too seriously.

I have found (through careful and bemused observance) that the women who take fashion and style too seriously start to go a bit crazy, and crazy looks good on a very, very select few. Cool, calm, and confident, however, looks good on pretty much anyone. You'll start to notice that the palpable air of cool confidence always comes from the corner of the room where the stylish women have gathered. They are not always the prettiest, the skinniest, or the wealthiest guests at the party. But they are often the savviest, because they know that none of these trifles (beauty, body, billfold) really matter. What does matter is that they are comfortable in their own skin. Watch these women, learn from these women, love yourself as these women love themselves, and you will find that style comes from adoring yourself enough to dress up for you and you alone. Because, in the end you are the only judge that really matters.

Style is a matter of finding out who you are and who you want to be in the world. I hope you choose to be fabulous, daring, fun, inspired, and yourself.

Everything you can imagine is real.

PABLO PICASSO

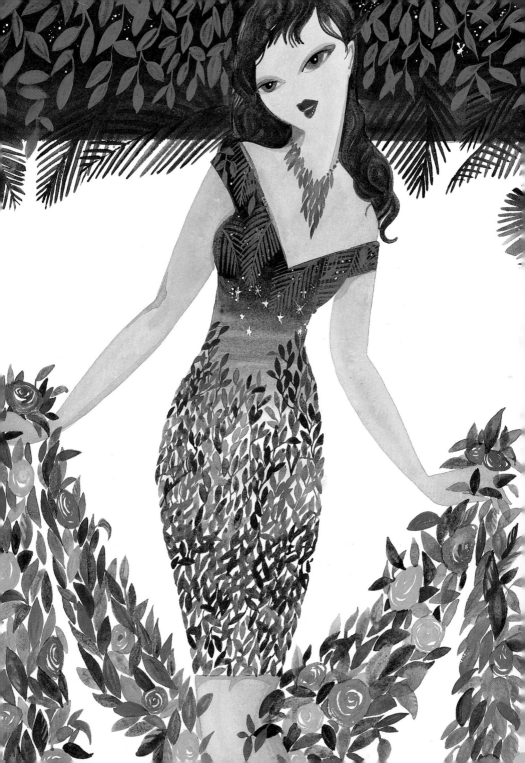

Acknowledgments

I WOULD LIKE TO THANK THOSE WHO MADE THIS BOOK POSSIBLE:

Rene Alegria, editor extraordinaire, for his endless patience and delayed deadlines.

HarperCollins for its incredibly professional team, most especially the talented Shubhani Sarkar.

Ruben Toledo, for the most amazing artwork—it is truly a dream come true to be in the same book with you.

My husband, David, and my son, Lucas: my favorite—and the most patient—men of all.

All of the designers (and the people behind them) for their gracious support and participation, including: Giorgio Armani, Christopher Bailey, Tory Burch, Roberto Cavalli, Francisco Costa, Victoire de Castellane, Oscar de la Renta, Domenico Dolce, Stefano Gabanna, John Galliano, Frida Giannini, Santiago Gonzalez, Carolina Herrera, Iman, Heidi Klum, Michael Kors, Reed Krakoff, Ralph Lauren, Christian Louboutin, Elle Macpherson, Gilles Mendel, Margherita Missoni, Zac Posen, Cameron Silver, Isabel Toledo, Diane von Furstenberg, Vera Wang, and Rachel Zoe.

All my friends at *Elle*, *Project Runway*, the Weinstein Company, Kym Canter, Jade Frampton, Malina Joseph, Erin Kaplan, Monica Haim, and Marissa Matteo.